WHOLESOME, SUPER GUTS

FOR WOMEN:

A COMPLETE GUIDE TO OPTIMAL DIGESTIVE AND HORMONAL HEALTH

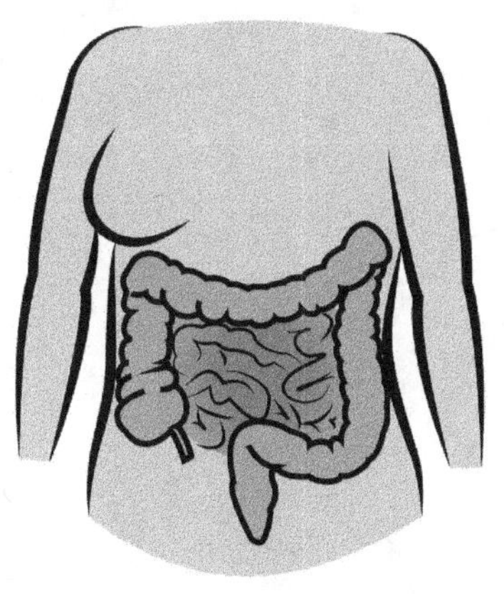

Elena Stephens

TABLE OF CONTENT

CHAPTER NINE - CRAFTING YOUR PERSONAL MEAL TIME.. **84**

CONCLUSION..**100**

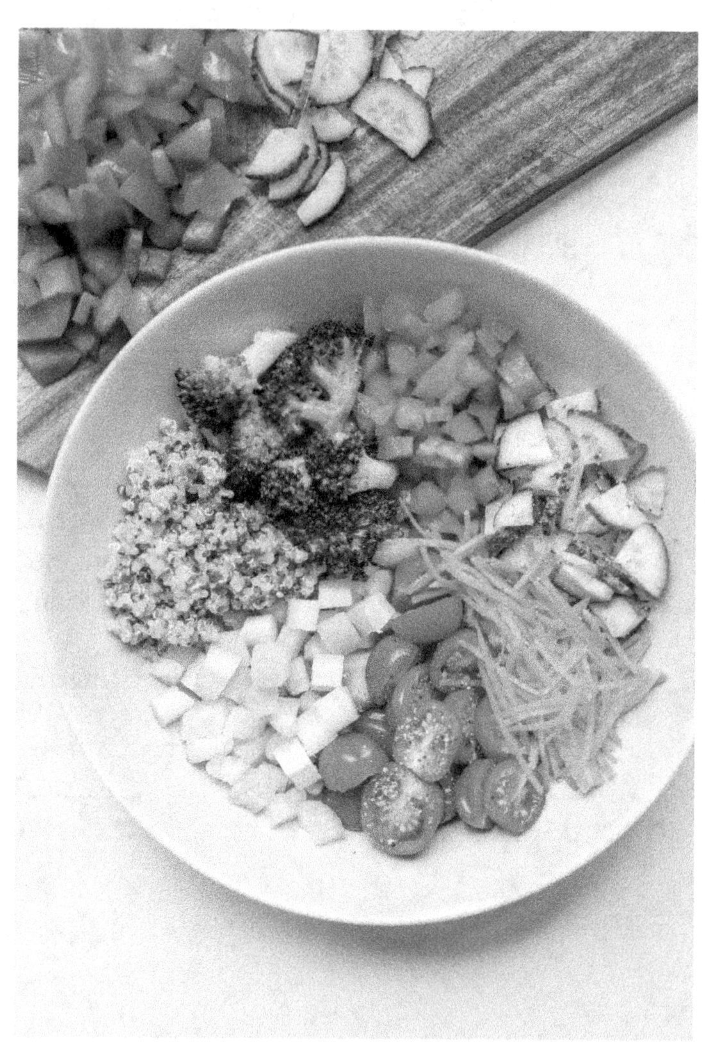

INTRODUCTION

Step into a world of vibrant health and vitality with 'Wholesome Super Guts for Women.' This comprehensive guide is your roadmap to unlocking the extraordinary power of gut health tailored specifically for the unique needs of women. As we navigate through the intricacies of the female body, this book transcends conventional wellness advice, offering a holistic approach that encompasses nutrition, lifestyle, and mindful practices. The journey begins with a deep dive into the fascinating interplay between gut health and the overall well-being of women. From the gut-brain connection to the profound impact of hormonal balance, each page is a revelation, empowering you with knowledge that transcends the ordinary.

Embrace a nourishing array of insights, from the significance of essential nutrients to the art of crafting gut-friendly recipes that cater to the distinct requirements of women at every stage of life. This guide doesn't just stop at information—it's a call to action. Explore the transformative potential of probiotics, prebiotics, and personalized meal plans, creating a foundation for a life marked by sustained energy, resilience, and joy. 'Wholesome Super Guts for Women' is not just a book; it's your companion on the path to becoming the healthiest, happiest version of yourself. Join us as we embark on this empowering journey to redefine well-being for women.

HOLISTIC HEALTH FOR WOMEN

Embracing Holistic Health for Women serves as the cornerstone of your transformative journey towards well-being. In this chapter, we embark on a holistic exploration of health that extends beyond the physical, delving into the interconnected realms of mental, emotional, and spiritual wellness. Recognizing the unique needs of women, we navigate the intricate dance between various aspects of life, understanding how they collectively contribute to a woman's overall vitality.

The chapter unfolds with a discussion on the significance of adopting a holistic approach to health. It emphasizes the interconnectedness of mind, body, and spirit, highlighting the profound impact each facet has on the others. As we weave through topics such as stress management, self-care, and mindfulness, the aim is to empower women to cultivate a balanced and harmonious life.

Through this journey, you'll discover practical tools, actionable insights, and empowering practices that transcend traditional health advice. The goal is not just to address symptoms but to nurture a comprehensive sense of well-being that radiates from within. "Embracing Holistic Health for Women" sets the stage for a transformative experience, inviting you to embark on a path towards true, sustainable health and happiness

THE SIGNIFICANCE OF GUT HEALTH

The significance of gut health extends far beyond mere digestion—it plays a crucial role in influencing various aspects of overall well-being. Here are key facets illustrating the importance of maintaining a healthy gut:

Digestive Efficiency: A well-functioning gut aids in the efficient breakdown and absorption of nutrients, ensuring the body receives the essential vitamins, minerals, and energy required for optimal functioning.

Immune Support: The gut is home to a significant portion of the immune system. A balanced and diverse microbiome helps defend against harmful pathogens, contributing to a robust immune response.

Hormonal Balance: The gut and endocrine system communicate bidirectionally. A healthy gut microbiome can influence the metabolism and regulation of hormones, contributing to hormonal balance throughout the body.

Mental Well-Being: The gut-brain axis, a bidirectional communication system between the gut and the brain, highlights the impact of gut health on mental health. A balanced gut microbiome is associated with better mood, cognitive function, and a lower risk of mental health disorders.

Inflammation Regulation: An imbalance in gut bacteria can lead to chronic inflammation, which is associated with various health issues, including autoimmune conditions, allergies, and chronic diseases.

Weight Management: The composition of the gut microbiome may influence metabolism and weight. An imbalanced gut flora has been linked to obesity and difficulties in weight management.

Energy Production: The gut microbiota plays a role in the fermentation of undigested carbohydrates, producing short-chain fatty acids (SCFAs), which serve as an energy source for the body.

Nutrient Synthesis: Certain beneficial bacteria in the gut contribute to the synthesis of vitamins, such as B vitamins and vitamin K, essential for various bodily functions.

Understanding and nurturing gut health through a balanced diet, probiotics, and mindful lifestyle choices is fundamental for promoting overall wellness and preventing a range of health issues.

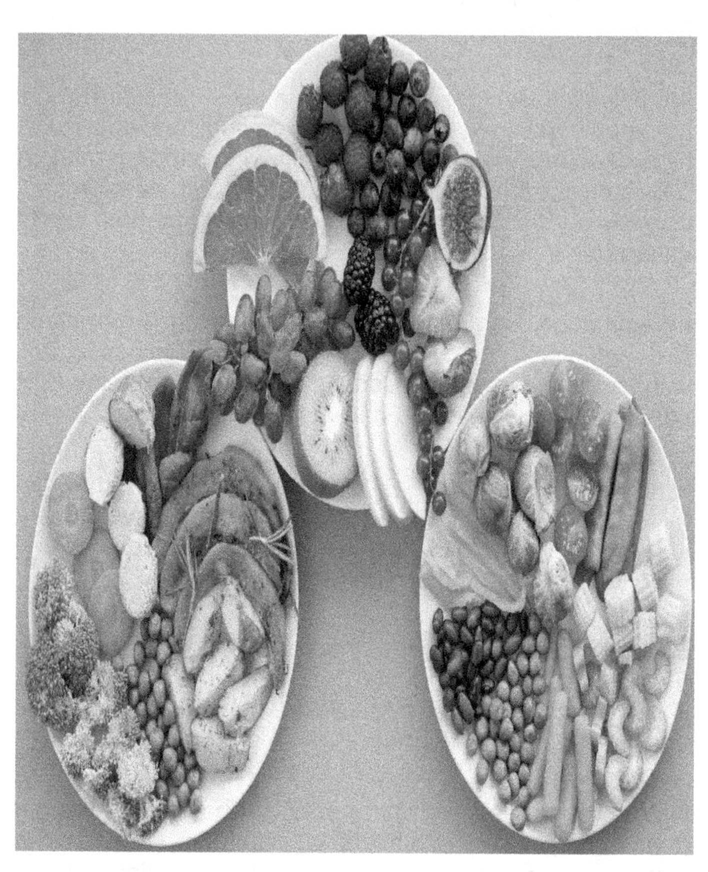

CHAPTER ONE - UNDERSTANDING THE GUT

Understanding the gut involves exploring the intricate system responsible for digesting food, absorbing nutrients, the complexity and the interconnectedness of its functions with various aspects of health and how it influences various aspects of overall health. Nurturing a healthy gut through a balanced diet, probiotics, and mindful practices contributes to overall well-being.

Here's an overview:

Gastrointestinal Tract: The gut, or gastrointestinal (GI) tract, spans from the mouth to the anus. It comprises organs such as the stomach, small intestine, large intestine (colon), and others, each with specific functions in the digestion and absorption process.

Microbiome: The gut is home to trillions of microorganisms, collectively known as the gut microbiome. This diverse ecosystem of bacteria, viruses, fungi, and other microbes plays a crucial role in maintaining balance and supporting various bodily functions.

Digestive Process: Digestion begins in the mouth with the breakdown of food by enzymes, followed by the stomach's acid and digestive enzymes. In the small intestine, nutrients are absorbed, and in the large intestine, water and electrolytes are reabsorbed, forming stool.

Absorption of Nutrients: The small intestine is a key site for nutrient absorption. Nutrients, including carbohydrates, proteins, fats, vitamins, and minerals, are absorbed into the bloodstream and transported to cells for energy and other functions.

Gut-Brain Axis: The bidirectional communication between the gut and the brain, known as the gut-brain axis, influences mood, emotions, and even cognitive function. The vagus nerve and the release of neurotransmitters contribute to this connection.

Hormonal Influence: The gut is involved in the production and regulation of hormones. For example, cells in the small intestine produce hormones that influence digestion and appetite.

Immune System Hub: A significant portion of the immune system resides in the gut-associated lymphoid tissue (GALT). The gut microbiome plays a vital role in training and modulating the immune system's response to pathogens.

Impact on Health: Imbalances in the gut microbiome have been linked to various health conditions, including digestive disorders, autoimmune diseases, mental health issues, and metabolic disorders.

Factors Influencing Gut Health: Diet, lifestyle, stress, antibiotics, and environmental factors can impact the composition and diversity of the gut microbiome, affecting overall gut health.

ANATOMY OF FEMALE DIGESTIVE SYSTEM

The anatomy of the female digestive system is a complex and highly organized structure responsible for the processing and absorption of nutrients. Here is an overview of the essential components:

Mouth:
The digestive process begins with the mouth, where food is ingested and broken down by chewing and mixed

with saliva, which contains digestive enzymes.

Esophagus:
A muscular tube that transports the chewed food from the mouth to the stomach through a coordinated process of muscle contractions known as peristalsis.

Stomach:
The stomach is a muscular organ that further breaks down food with gastric juices, including hydrochloric acid and enzymes, forming a semi-liquid substance known as chyme.

Small Intestine:
Divided into three parts (duodenum, jejunum, and ileum), the small intestine is where the majority of nutrient absorption occurs. Nutrient absorption and breakdown are aided by pancreatic enzymes and liver bile.

Liver:
Produces bile, which emulsifies lipids and facilitates their absorption and digestion. The liver also plays a role in processing nutrients and detoxifying the blood.

Gallbladder:
Stores and releases bile produced by the liver. Bile is released into the small intestine to aid in the digestion and absorption of fats.

Pancreas:
Produces digestive enzymes that are released into the small intestine to further break down carbohydrates, proteins, and fats.

Large Intestine (Colon):
forms feces by absorbing water and electrolytes from the leftover undigested meal. The colon also houses a significant portion of the gut microbiome, which aids in

the fermentation of indigestible carbohydrates.

Rectum:
The final portion of the digestive tract where feces are stored before being eliminated.
Anus:
the orifice where feces exit the body during bowel motions at the end of the digestive tract.

The female digestive system shares commonalities with the male digestive system, but it also undergoes unique challenges, such as hormonal fluctuations that can influence digestion. Understanding the anatomy of the female digestive system is essential for maintaining overall health and addressing specific digestive concerns that may arise.

THE GUT-BRAIN CONNECTION

The gut-brain connection refers to the bidirectional communication between the gastrointestinal (GI) tract and the central nervous system, particularly the brain. This intricate interaction involves a complex network of neural, hormonal, and immunological signals, and it plays a crucial role in influencing various aspects of physical and mental well-being. Here are key aspects of the gut-brain connection:

Vagus Nerve:
The vagus nerve is a major player in the gut-brain axis, connecting the brainstem to the gut. It facilitates the transmission of signals in both directions, allowing the brain to influence gut function and vice versa.

Neurotransmitters:
The gut produces and houses a significant amount of neurotransmitters, including serotonin and dopamine. These chemicals, traditionally associated with mood regulation, have a profound impact on mental health and

can influence emotions and cognition.

Hormones:
Hormones released in the gut, such as ghrelin and leptin, influence appetite and metabolism. The brain receives signals from these hormones, affecting feelings of hunger, satiety, and energy balance.
Microbiome Influence:
The gut microbiome, a diverse community of microorganisms residing in the digestive tract, produces metabolites that can influence neural function and communication. Changes in the microbiome composition have been linked to alterations in mood and behavior.

Immune System Modulation:
The gut is a significant component of the immune system, and immune cells in the gut can release signaling molecules that affect the brain. Inflammatory responses in the gut may impact mood and cognitive function.

Stress Response:
Stress, whether acute or chronic, can affect gut function and alter the balance of the gut microbiome. Conversely, disturbances in the gut can contribute to stress responses.

Impact on Mental Health:
Imbalances in the gut-brain axis have been associated with various mental health conditions, including anxiety, depression, and certain neurological disorders.

Gut Health and Cognitive Function:
Emerging research suggests that maintaining a healthy gut may contribute to better cognitive function and a reduced risk of neurodegenerative diseases.

Understanding and nurturing the gut-brain connection is integral to promoting overall well-being. Lifestyle factors such as diet, stress management, and probiotic intake can positively influence this axis, highlighting the importance of a holistic approach to health that considers the interconnectedness of the gut and the brain.

HORMONAL INFLUENCES ON GUT HEALTH

Hormonal influences play a significant role in maintaining the delicate balance of the gut, affecting various aspects of digestive function and overall gut health. Here are key hormonal factors that impact the gastrointestinal (GI) system:

Gastrin:
Produced in the stomach, gastrin stimulates the secretion of gastric acid, promoting digestion. An imbalance in gastrin levels can contribute to acid-related conditions, such as gastritis or peptic ulcers.

Ghrelin:
Often referred to as the "hunger hormone," ghrelin is produced in the stomach and signals the brain to stimulate appetite. Fluctuations in ghrelin levels can influence feelings of hunger and satiety.

Leptin:
Secreted by fat cells, leptin acts as an appetite suppressor, signaling to the brain when the body has sufficient energy stores. Leptin resistance, where the brain doesn't respond adequately to leptin, may contribute to overeating and obesity.

Insulin:
While primarily associated with blood sugar regulation, insulin can indirectly influence gut health. Insulin resistance, often seen in conditions like type 2 diabetes, has been linked to alterations in gut microbiota.

Cortisol:
Released in response to stress, cortisol can affect

various aspects of digestion. Chronic stress and elevated cortisol levels may contribute to conditions like irritable bowel syndrome (IBS) and gastrointestinal discomfort.

Estrogen and Progesterone:
These sex hormones can influence gut motility and function. Fluctuations in estrogen and progesterone levels during the menstrual cycle can contribute to changes in bowel habits, and hormonal shifts during menopause may impact gut health.

Thyroid Hormones (T3 and T4):
Thyroid hormones influence metabolism, and imbalances, such as hypothyroidism or hyperthyroidism, can lead to changes in bowel function. Hypothyroidism, for example, is associated with constipation.

Serotonin:
Primarily known as a neurotransmitter, serotonin is also produced in the gut. It regulates bowel movements, and alterations in serotonin levels are linked to conditions like irritable bowel syndrome (IBS).

Peptide YY (PYY):
Released in the small intestine, PYY helps regulate appetite and slows down the movement of food through the digestive tract, contributing to feelings of fullness.

Understanding the intricate interplay between hormones and gut health is crucial for addressing digestive issues and promoting overall well-being. Lifestyle factors, including a balanced diet, regular exercise, and stress management, can positively influence hormonal balance and support optimal gut function.

CHAPTER TWO - NOURISHING NUTRIENTS

Nourishing nutrients refers to essential substances found in food that provide the body with the energy and building blocks required for optimal functioning. These nutrients are vital for various physiological processes, supporting overall health and well-being. Here are key categories of nourishing nutrients:

A balanced and varied diet that incorporates a spectrum of these nourishing nutrients is fundamental for promoting optimal health, supporting growth, and preventing nutrient deficiencies. Dietary choices should align with individual needs, taking into account factors such as age, sex, activity level, and specific health goals.

ESSENTIAL VITAMINS AND MINERALS FOR WOMEN

Women have unique nutritional needs, and ensuring an adequate intake of essential vitamins and minerals is crucial for overall health and well-being. Here are key vitamins and minerals that play a significant role in women's health:

1. Folate (Vitamin B9):
Importance: Critical for fetal development during pregnancy, supports DNA synthesis, and helps prevent neural tube defects.

Sources: Leafy greens, legumes, fortified cereals, and citrus fruits.

2. Iron:
Importance: Vital for the formation of hemoglobin and preventing iron-deficiency anemia, especially during

menstruation and pregnancy.

Sources: Red meat, poultry, fish, fortified cereals, beans, and leafy greens.

3. Calcium:
Importance: Essential for bone health, nerve function, and muscle contraction.

Sources: Dairy products, leafy greens, fortified plant-based milk, and fish with edible bones.

4. Vitamin D:
Importance: Facilitates calcium absorption, supports bone health, and plays a role in immune function.

Sources: Sunlight exposure, fatty fish, fortified dairy or plant-based milk, and egg yolks.

5. Vitamin K:
Importance: Supports blood clotting and bone health.

Sources: Leafy greens (kale, spinach), broccoli, and soybean oil.

6. Magnesium:
Importance: Supports muscle and nerve function, bone health, and energy production.

Sources: Nuts, seeds, whole grains, leafy greens, and legumes.

7. Vitamin C:
Importance: Acts as an antioxidant, supports immune function, and aids in collagen synthesis.

Sources: Citrus fruits, strawberries, bell peppers, and broccoli.

8. Vitamin E:
Importance: Antioxidant that protects cells from damage, supports skin health, and may have cardiovascular benefits.

Sources: Nuts, seeds, spinach, and vegetable oils.

9. B Vitamins (B6, B12, Riboflavin):
Importance: Essential for energy metabolism, red blood cell formation, and neurological health.

Sources: Poultry, fish, eggs, dairy, and fortified cereals.

10. Zinc:
Importance: Supports immune function, wound healing, and reproductive health.

Sources: Meat, dairy, nuts, seeds, and legumes.

Meeting these nutritional needs through a well-balanced diet is ideal. However, certain life stages, dietary preferences, or health conditions may necessitate supplementation. Women should consult with healthcare professionals to ensure they are meeting their specific nutrient requirements for optimal health.

THE ROLE OF FIBER IN GUT WELLNESS

Dietary fiber plays a crucial role in promoting gut wellness and supporting overall digestive health. Here are key aspects of the role of fiber in maintaining a healthy gut:

1. Digestive Regularity:
Bulk Formation: Fiber adds bulk to the stool, promoting regular bowel movements and preventing constipation. It absorbs water, softening the stool and facilitating its passage through the digestive tract.

2. Gut Microbiota Health:
Prebiotic Effect: Certain types of fiber, known as prebiotics, serve as food for beneficial gut bacteria. By promoting the growth of these bacteria, fiber contributes to a balanced and diverse gut microbiota, which is essential for overall health.

3. Weight Management:
Satiety: High-fiber foods help create a feeling of fullness, reducing overall calorie intake and supporting weight management.

4. Blood Sugar Regulation:
Slow Carbohydrate Absorption: Soluble fiber can slow down the absorption of sugar, helping to regulate blood glucose levels. This is particularly beneficial for individuals with diabetes or those at risk of developing insulin resistance.

5. Heart Health:
Cholesterol Reduction: Soluble fiber, such as that found in oats and beans, can help lower cholesterol levels by binding to cholesterol and removing it from the body.

6. Prevention of Diverticulosis:
Increased Bulk: Adequate fiber intake can prevent the formation of small pouches in the colon (diverticula) that may lead to diverticulosis.

7. Colon Health:
Reduced Risk of Colorectal Cancer: High-fiber diets are associated with a lower risk of developing colorectal cancer. Fiber may help protect against this type of cancer by promoting regular bowel movements and

providing beneficial compounds to the colon.

8. Inflammatory Bowel Diseases (IBD):
Symptom Management: For individuals with inflammatory bowel diseases like Crohn's disease or ulcerative colitis, soluble fiber may help manage symptoms by providing a source of nutrition that is gentler on the digestive tract.

9. Detoxification:
Binding Toxins: Certain fibers, particularly insoluble fiber found in vegetables and whole grains, can bind to toxins and facilitate their excretion from the body.

10. Prevention of Hemorrhoids:
Softening Stool: Fiber helps maintain soft, bulky stool, reducing the risk of straining during bowel movements and preventing the development of hemorrhoids.

To harness the benefits of fiber for gut wellness, it is important to consume a variety of fiber-rich foods, including fruits, vegetables, whole grains, legumes, and nuts. It's recommended to gradually increase fiber intake and stay adequately hydrated to optimize its effects on digestion and gut health.

OMEGA-3 FATTY ACIDS FOR HORMONAL BALANCE

Omega-3 fatty acids play a significant role in promoting hormonal balance and overall well-being. These essential fats, particularly eicosapentaenoic acid (EPA) and docosahexaenoic acid (DHA), are primarily found in fatty fish, algae, and certain plant sources. Here's how omega-3 fatty acids contribute to hormonal health:

1. Anti-Inflammatory Effects:
Omega-3s are known for their anti-inflammatory properties. Chronic inflammation can disrupt hormonal

balance and contribute to conditions such as insulin resistance. By reducing inflammation, omega-3s may help maintain hormonal equilibrium.

2. Support for Endocrine System:
The endocrine system, responsible for hormone production and regulation, benefits from omega-3s. These fatty acids are involved in the structure and function of cell membranes, influencing the responsiveness of cells to hormones.

3. Influence on Insulin Sensitivity:
Omega-3s may improve insulin sensitivity, helping to regulate blood sugar levels. This can be particularly beneficial for women with conditions like polycystic ovary syndrome (PCOS), where insulin resistance is common.

4. Hormones in Menstrual Cycle:
Omega-3s may contribute to a more balanced menstrual cycle by influencing the production and activity of hormones involved in the menstrual process, such as prostaglandins.

5. Hormonal Health During Pregnancy:
DHA, a type of omega-3, is crucial for the development of the fetal brain and nervous system during pregnancy. Adequate omega-3 intake is associated with a lower risk of preterm birth and may contribute to hormonal balance during this critical period.

6. Mood Regulation:
Mood regulation and mental health are linked to Omega-3s. They may have a positive impact on neurotransmitters and hormones that influence mood, such as serotonin and dopamine.

7. Reduction of PMS Symptoms:
Some studies suggest that omega-3 supplementation may help alleviate symptoms of premenstrual syndrome (PMS), including mood swings, bloating, and breast

tenderness.

8. Cardiovascular Health:
Heart health is closely connected to hormonal balance. Omega-3s contribute to cardiovascular health, influencing hormones related to blood pressure regulation and blood vessel function.

9. Anti-Aging Benefits:
Omega-3s may contribute to healthy skin by supporting the production of hormones that play a role in skin integrity. This may have anti-aging effects on the skin.
10. Postmenopausal Health:

Omega-3s may provide benefits for postmenopausal women by supporting cardiovascular health, reducing inflammation, and potentially alleviating certain symptoms associated with hormonal changes.

Incorporating omega-3-rich foods such as fatty fish (salmon, mackerel, sardines), flaxseeds, chia seeds, and walnuts into the diet or considering omega-3 supplements can contribute to hormonal balance and support overall health. As with any dietary change or supplementation, it's advisable to consult with a healthcare professional for personalized advice based on individual health needs.

CHAPTER THREE - WHOLESOME NUTRITION FOR WOMEN.

Wholesome nutrition for women involves adopting a balanced and nutrient-dense diet that addresses the unique needs of the female body at different life stages. Here are key principles for achieving wholesome nutrition for women:

Balanced Macronutrients: Ensure a balanced intake of macronutrients carbohydrates, proteins, and fats. Opt for whole grains, lean proteins (such as poultry, fish, beans, and legumes), and healthy fats from sources like avocados, nuts, and olive oil.

Adequate Calcium Intake: Calcium is crucial for bone health, especially for women who are more prone to osteoporosis. Include dairy products, fortified plant-based milk, leafy greens, and fish with edible bones in your diet.

Iron-Rich Foods: Women, particularly during menstruation and pregnancy, need adequate iron to prevent anemia. Include iron-rich foods such as lean meats, beans, lentils, and fortified cereals in your meals.

Folate-Rich Foods: Folate is essential for reproductive health and is particularly important during pregnancy. Consume folate-rich foods such as leafy greens, citrus fruits, legumes, and fortified grains.

Omega-3 Fatty Acids: Support hormonal balance and cardiovascular health by including sources of omega-3 fatty acids, such as fatty fish (salmon, mackerel), flaxseeds, chia seeds, and walnuts.

Fiber-Rich Diet: Prioritize fiber for digestive health and weight management. Incorporate whole grains, fruits, vegetables, legumes, and nuts to ensure an ample intake of dietary fiber.

Antioxidant-Rich Foods: Combat oxidative stress by including a variety of colorful fruits and vegetables in your diet. Berries, tomatoes, spinach, and other antioxidant-rich foods contribute to overall health.

Hydration: Stay hydrated, because water is crucial for digestion and nutrient absorption., and overall bodily functions. Aim to consume water, herbal teas, and hydrating foods throughout the day.

Lean Protein Sources: Choose lean protein sources to support muscle health and provide a steady supply of amino acids. Incorporate poultry, fish, tofu, and plant-based protein options into your meals.

Mindful Eating: Pay attention to hunger and fullness indicators to cultivate mindful eating skills. Avoid restrictive diets and focus on nourishing your body with a variety of nutrient-dense foods.

Adapt to Life Stages: Tailor your nutrition to different life stages, including adolescence, reproductive years, pregnancy, postpartum, and menopause. Consult with healthcare professionals for personalized guidance during specific life transitions.

Limit Processed Foods and Added Sugars: Reduce the consumption of processed foods and foods high in added sugars. Focus on whole, minimally processed foods to maximize nutritional benefits.

Adopting a wholesome approach to nutrition involves creating a sustainable and enjoyable eating pattern that supports overall health and well-being. It's advisable to consult with a registered dietitian or healthcare professional to develop a personalized nutrition plan based on individual needs and goals.

BUILDING A BALANCED PLATE

Building a balanced plate involves selecting a variety of nutrient-dense foods to ensure you receive essential nutrients in appropriate proportions. Here's a guide to creating a well-balanced plate:

Fill Half Your Plate with Vegetables: Choose a colorful array of vegetables. They are rich in antioxidants, minerals, fiber, and vitamins. Include leafy greens, cruciferous vegetables, bell peppers, tomatoes, and carrots.

Add Lean Protein: Include a source of lean protein to support muscle health and keep you feeling satisfied. Options include poultry, fish, tofu, legumes, beans, lentils, and lean cuts of meat.

Incorporate Whole Grains: Choose whole grains for complex carbohydrates, fiber, and various nutrients. Opt for brown rice, quinoa, whole wheat pasta, barley, or oats instead of refined grains.

Include Healthy Fats: Integrate sources of healthy fats to support heart health and aid in the absorption of fat-soluble vitamins. Examples include avocados, nuts, seeds, olive oil, and fatty fish like salmon.

Portion Control: Be mindful of portion sizes to avoid overeating. Use smaller plates and bowls, and listen to your body's hunger and fullness cues.

Diversify Your Protein Sources: Vary your protein sources to ensure a mix of essential amino acids. Incorporate plant-based proteins like beans, lentils, and tofu alongside animal-based proteins.

Minimize Added Sugars and Processed Foods: Limit the intake of foods high in added sugars and processed items. Focus on whole, minimally processed foods to maximize nutritional benefits.

Hydrate with Water: Stay hydrated by consuming water throughout the day. Minimize sugary beverages and consider herbal teas or infused water for added flavor.

Consider Nutrient Density: Choose nutrient-dense foods that provide a high amount of vitamins and minerals relative to their calorie content. This includes a variety of fruits, vegetables, whole grains, and lean proteins.

Mindful Eating: Savor each bite, pay attention to hunger and fullness signs, and keep distractions to a minimum when eating.

Example of a Balanced Plate:

Half the Plate: Colorful vegetables like broccoli, bell peppers, and carrots.

- Quarter of the Plate: Grilled chicken breast or tofu for protein.
- Quarter of the Plate: Quinoa or brown rice for whole grains.
- A Drizzle of Healthy Fat: Olive oil dressing on the vegetables or a sprinkle of nuts/seeds.

Adjustments for Specific Diets or Dietary Restrictions:

- Consider individual dietary needs, such as vegetarian or vegan preferences, gluten-free requirements, or specific health conditions. Adjust the plate composition accordingly.

Building a balanced plate is a flexible approach that allows for creativity and adaptation based on personal preferences and nutritional requirements. Remember to consult with a registered dietitian or healthcare professional for personalized guidance based on your specific needs and goals.

SUPER FOODS FOR FEMALE VITALITY AND HORMONAL HEALTH

While there isn't a single "superfood" that can address all aspects of female vitality and maintaining of hormonal balance, incorporating a variety of nutrient-dense foods into the diet can provide essential nutrients and support overall well-being. Here are some superfoods for female vitality:

Salmon (or other Fatty Fish): Rich in omega-3 fatty acids, salmon supports heart health, reduces inflammation, and may contribute to hormonal balance.

Berries (Blueberries, Strawberries, etc.): Packed with antioxidants, vitamins, and fiber, berries offer numerous health benefits, including support for skin health and cognitive function.

Dark Leafy Greens (Spinach, Kale, Swiss Chard): High in iron, calcium, and vitamins, dark leafy greens are essential for bone health, energy production, and overall vitality.

Avocado: A source of healthy monounsaturated fats, avocados provide energy and support hormonal health. They also contain various vitamins and minerals.

Greek Yogurt: Rich in protein and probiotics, Greek yogurt promotes gut health, supports digestion, and provides a source of calcium for bone health.

Quinoa: A nutrient-dense whole grain, quinoa is rich in protein, fiber, and essential minerals, making it an excellent choice for sustained energy.

Sweet Potatoes: High in vitamins, particularly vitamin A, sweet potatoes support skin health, immune function, and vision.

Nuts and Seeds (Almonds, Chia Seeds, Flaxseeds): Packed with healthy fats, protein, and essential nutrients, nuts and seeds contribute to heart health and provide sustained energy.

Broccoli: A cruciferous vegetable, broccoli contains vitamins, minerals, and antioxidants that support immune health and may have anti-inflammatory properties.

Beans and Legumes: Rich in fiber, protein, and various nutrients, beans and legumes support digestive health, provide sustained energy, and contribute to overall vitality.

Turmeric: Known for its anti-inflammatory properties, turmeric contains curcumin, which may help manage inflammation and support joint health.

Eggs: A complete protein source, eggs provide essential amino acids, vitamins, and minerals. They support muscle health, energy production, and overall well-being.

Flaxseeds: High in omega-3 fatty acids, fiber, and lignans, flaxseeds contribute to heart health, hormonal balance, and digestive well-being.

Green Tea: Rich in antioxidants and known for its potential health benefits, green tea may support metabolism, cognitive function, and overall vitality.

Beets: Packed with vitamins, minerals, and antioxidants, beets support cardiovascular health, may enhance exercise performance, and contribute to overall vitality.

Chia Seeds: Rich in omega-3 fatty acids, fiber, and protein, chia seeds may help balance blood sugar levels and support hormonal health.

Eggs: A good source of high-quality protein and various vitamins, eggs provide nutrients essential for hormone synthesis.

Wild Yam: Contains compounds that are precursors to progesterone and is traditionally believed to support hormonal balance, especially in women.

Pomegranates: Rich in antioxidants, pomegranates may have anti-inflammatory effects and support hormonal health.

Salmon: Along with being a great source of omega-3s, salmon contains vitamin D, which is important for hormone regulation.

Coconut Oil: Contains medium-chain triglycerides (MCTs), which may support hormone production and balance

Remember, a balanced and varied diet that includes a wide range of nutrient-dense foods is essential for female vitality and hormonal health support. Additionally, individual dietary needs may vary, and it's advisable to consult with a registered dietitian or healthcare professional for personalized nutrition advice based on specific health goals and conditions.

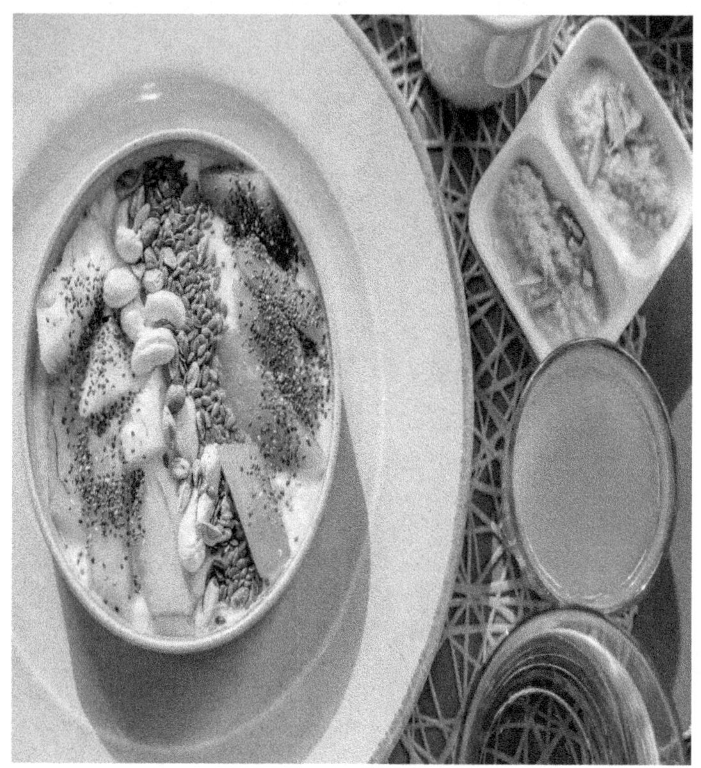

CHAPTER FOUR - GUT-FRIENDLY RECIPES

Creating gut-friendly recipes involves incorporating foods that support digestive health and promote a balanced gut microbiome. These recipes should incorporate fiber, fermented foods, and ingredients rich in prebiotics and probiotics—key elements for gut health.

BREAKFAST BOOSTERS

Starting your day with gut-friendly breakfast options can set a positive tone for your digestive health. Here are two breakfast booster recipes that focus on ingredients known for their gut-friendly properties:

1. Overnight Chia Seed Pudding:

Ingredients:
- 3 tablespoons chia seeds
- 1 cup almond milk (or any preferred milk)
- 1/2 teaspoon vanilla extract
- 1 tablespoon honey or maple syrup
- Fresh berries for topping

Instructions:
In a bowl, combine chia seeds, almond milk, vanilla extract, and honey. Stir well.
Cover the bowl and refrigerate overnight, or for at least 4 hours, until the mixture thickens to a pudding consistency.
Before serving, give the mixture a good stir.
Top with fresh berries and enjoy this fiber-rich, probiotic-free breakfast.

2. Gut-Healing Smoothie Bowl:
Ingredients:
- 1 cup Greek yogurt (or dairy-free alternative)
- 1/2 cup frozen pineapple chunks
- 1/2 cup mango chunks
- 1 small banana
- 1 tablespoon ground flaxseeds
- 1 tablespoon almond butter
- Toppings: Granola, sliced almonds, and a drizzle of honey

Instructions:

In a blender, combine Greek yogurt, frozen pineapple, mango, banana, flaxseeds, and almond butter.
Blend until smooth and creamy.
Pour the smoothie into a bowl and add your favorite toppings like granola, sliced almonds, and a drizzle of honey.
Enjoy this nutrient-packed, probiotic-rich breakfast bowl.

Creating gut-friendly recipes involves incorporating foods that support digestive health and promote a balanced gut microbiome. Here are two recipes that focus on ingredients known for their gut-friendly properties:

3. Quinoa and Vegetable Buddha Bowl:

Ingredients:
- 1 cup cooked quinoa
- 1 cup mixed vegetables (e.g., broccoli, bell peppers, carrots)
- 1 cup leafy greens (e.g., kale, spinach)
- 1/2 cup sauerkraut (fermented cabbage)
- 1/4 cup sliced almonds
- 1 tablespoon olive oil
- 1 tablespoon lemon juice
- Salt and pepper to taste

Instructions:
Steam or stir-fry the mixed vegetables until they are tender but still vibrant.

In a bowl, combine cooked quinoa, steamed vegetables, leafy greens, sauerkraut, and sliced almonds.

In a small bowl, whisk together olive oil, lemon juice, salt, and pepper to create a simple dressing.

Drizzle the dressing over the Buddha bowl and toss gently to combine.

Serve immediately and enjoy this nutrient-packed, gut-friendly bowl.

These breakfast recipes incorporate chia seeds, yogurt, and other gut-friendly ingredients to provide a combination of fiber, probiotics, and prebiotics. Remember to stay hydrated and personalize these recipes according to your taste preferences and dietary needs for a delicious and digestive-friendly start to your day.

LUNCHES FOR GUT WELLNESS

Promoting gut wellness through your lunch choices involves incorporating foods that support digestion, provide beneficial nutrients, and contribute to a balanced microbiome. Here are two lunch ideas for gut wellness:

1. Quinoa and Chickpea Salad:

Ingredients:
- 1 cup cooked quinoa
- 1 cup canned chickpeas, drained and rinsed
- 1 cucumber, diced
- 1 cup cherry tomatoes, halved

- 1/4 cup red onion, finely chopped
- 1/4 cup feta cheese, crumbled
- 2 tablespoons extra-virgin olive oil
- 1 tablespoon lemon juice
- 1 teaspoon dried oregano
- Salt and pepper to taste
- Fresh parsley for garnish

Instructions:

In a large bowl, combine quinoa, chickpeas, cucumber, cherry tomatoes, red onion, and feta cheese.

In a small bowl, whisk together olive oil, lemon juice, dried oregano, salt, and pepper to create a dressing.

Add the dressing over the salad and mix until well combined.

Garnish with fresh parsley.

Serve as a refreshing and fiber-rich lunch option.

2. Gut-Healing Miso Soup with Tofu and Vegetables:

Ingredients:
- 4 cups vegetable broth
- 2 tablespoons miso paste
- 1 cup tofu, cubed
- 1 cup broccoli florets
- 1 carrot, julienned
- 1 cup spinach leaves
- 2 green onions, sliced
- 1 tablespoon soy sauce
- 1 teaspoon sesame oil
- Cooked brown rice or quinoa (optional)

Instructions:

In a pot, heat vegetable broth until warm but not boiling.

In a small bowl, dissolve miso paste in a bit of warm broth, then add it back to the pot.

Add tofu, broccoli, and carrot to the pot and simmer until vegetables are tender.
Stir in spinach, green onions, soy sauce, and sesame oil.
Let the soup simmer for a few more minutes.
Serve as is or over a bed of cooked brown rice or quinoa.

These lunch ideas incorporate fiber-rich foods, fermented ingredients (such as miso), and a variety of vegetables to support gut health. Remember to stay hydrated and make adjustments based on individual preferences and dietary needs. If you have specific digestive concerns, it's advisable to consult with a healthcare professional or a registered dietitian for personalized advice.

DINNER DELIGHTS

Dinner is an excellent opportunity to continue supporting gut wellness through nourishing and balanced choices. Here are two dinner ideas that focus on ingredients beneficial for digestive health:

1. Grilled Salmon with Quinoa and Roasted Vegetables:

Ingredients:
- 1 salmon filet
- 1 cup cooked quinoa
- 1 cup mixed vegetables (e.g., zucchini, bell peppers, cherry tomatoes)
- 1 tablespoon olive oil
- 1 lemon (for zest and juice)
- 1 teaspoon dried herbs (such as thyme or rosemary)
- Salt and pepper to taste

Instructions:

Preheat the oven to 400°F (200°C).
Place the salmon filet on a baking sheet lined with parchment paper.
In a bowl, toss the mixed vegetables with olive oil, lemon zest, dried herbs, salt, and pepper.
Arrange the veggies on the baking sheet in a circle around the salmon.
Bake for 15 to 20 minutes, or until the veggies are soft and the salmon is cooked through, in a preheated oven.
Serve the grilled salmon on a bed of cooked quinoa, with the roasted vegetables on the side.
Squeeze fresh lemon juice on the dish before serving.

2. Gut-Healing Lentil Soup:

Ingredients:

- 1 cup dry green or brown lentils, rinsed
- 1 onion, chopped
- 2 carrots, diced
- 2 celery stalks, chopped
- 3 cloves garlic, minced
- 1 can (14 oz) diced tomatoes
- 6 cups vegetable broth
- 1 teaspoon ground cumin
- 1 teaspoon ground coriander
- 1/2 teaspoon turmeric
- Salt and pepper to taste
- Fresh cilantro or parsley for garnish

Instructions:

In a large pot, sauté the chopped onion, carrots, and celery in olive oil until softened.
Add minced garlic, cumin, coriander, and turmeric. Stir for another minute.
Pour in the vegetable broth, lentils, and diced tomatoes with their juice.

Bring the soup to a boil, then reduce the heat and let it simmer for about 25-30 minutes or until lentils are tender.
Season with salt and pepper to taste.
Serve hot, garnished with fresh cilantro or parsley.

These dinner recipes emphasize lean proteins, fiber-rich ingredients, and a variety of vegetables, all of which contribute to a well-balanced and gut-friendly meal.

SNACKS FOR SUSTAINED ENERGY

Certainly! Snacks that provide a combination of complex carbohydrates, healthy fats, and protein can help sustain energy levels throughout the day. Here are some snack ideas for sustained energy:

1. Apple Slices with Nut Butter: Spread almond butter or peanut butter on apple slices for a tasty combination of fiber, healthy fats, and protein.

2. Greek Yogurt Parfait: Layer Greek yogurt with fresh berries, a drizzle of honey, and granola for a balance of protein, vitamins, and complex carbohydrates.

3. Trail Mix: Create your own trail mix with a mix of nuts, seeds, dried fruits, and a sprinkle of dark chocolate for a blend of healthy fats, protein, and carbohydrates.

4. Hummus with Veggie Sticks: Dip carrot, cucumber, and bell pepper sticks into hummus. The combination of fiber and protein helps to keep you full and satisfied.

5. Whole Grain Crackers with Cheese: Choose whole grain crackers and pair them with cheese for a combination of complex carbohydrates and protein.

6. Oatmeal Energy Bites: Make energy bites using rolled oats, nut butter, honey, and add-ins like chia seeds or dried fruit. These provide a mix of fiber and healthy fats.

7. Edamame: Enjoy a handful of steamed edamame sprinkled with sea salt for a protein-packed, satisfying snack.

8. Smoothie with Spinach and Banana: Blend a smoothie with spinach, banana, Greek yogurt, and a scoop of protein powder for a nutrient-rich and energizing drink.

9. Rice Cake with Avocado: Top a rice cake with mashed avocado, a sprinkle of sea salt, and a drizzle of olive oil for a balanced snack.

10. Cottage Cheese With Pineapple : Combine cottage cheese with fresh pineapple chunks for a mix of protein and natural sweetness

11. Chia Pudding: Make chia pudding with almond milk, chia seed and a touch of honey. Top with berries.

12. Hard Boiled Eggs: Hard-boil eggs and sprinkle them with a pinch of salt and pepper for a portable and protein-rich snack.

Cultivating mindful eating habits can lead to a more positive and intentional relationship with food, promoting better digestion and overall well-being. Start with small steps and gradually incorporate these practices into your meals for a more mindful eating experience.

CHAPTER FIVE - MINDFUL EATING PRACTICES

Mindful eating is a practice that involves paying full attention to the experience of eating, including the tastes, smells, textures, and sensations of the food. It encourages a non-judgmental awareness of your thoughts and feelings about food. Here are some mindful eating practices to incorporate into your routine:

Eat Without Distractions: Turn off the TV, put away your phone, and avoid other distractions while eating. Focus solely on the act of eating and the sensory experience of each bite.

Appreciate Your Food: Take a moment to visually appreciate your meal. Notice the colors, textures, and arrangement of the food on your plate.

Use All Your Senses: Engage all your senses in the eating experience. Smell the aromas, savor the flavors, feel the textures, and listen to the sounds as you chew.

Chew Slowly and Thoroughly: Chew your food slowly and thoroughly. This not only improves digestion, but also allows you to completely experience and appreciate the flavors.

Pause Between Bites: Put your utensils down between bites. This simple act encourages a slower pace of eating and gives you time to check in with your hunger and fullness cues.

Express Gratitude: Before you begin eating, take a moment to express gratitude for the food in front of you. Reflect on where it came from and the effort involved in bringing it to your plate.

Listen to Your Hunger Cues: Pay attention to your body's hunger and fullness signals. Eat when you're hungry and stop when you're satisfied, not overly full.

Be Mindful of Portion Sizes: Consider portion sizes that align with your body's needs. Use smaller plates to help control portions and prevent overeating.

Identify Emotional Triggers: Notice if you're eating due to emotions or external cues rather than hunger. Mindful eating involves being aware of emotional eating patterns.

Practice Gratitude: Reflect on the meal after finishing. Acknowledge the nourishment it provided and any positive feelings associated with the experience.

Savor Each Bite: Take the time to savor each bite. Avoid rushing through your meal and focus on the present moment.

Eat Regularly And Balanced: Maintain regular meal time and aim for balanced, nutritious meals to support overall well-being.

ACT OF INTUITIVE EATING

Intuitive eating is an approach to eating that encourages listening to your body's signals, honoring hunger and fullness, and cultivating a healthy relationship with food. Here are the key acts of intuitive eating:

Listening to Hunger and Fullness: Pay attention to your body's hunger cues. Eat when you're hungry and stop when you're satisfied. Allow your internal signals to guide your eating patterns.

Eating for Physical, Not Emotional Reasons: Distinguish between physical hunger and emotional cues. Eat to satisfy physical hunger rather than using food as a response to stress, boredom, or other emotions.

Making Peace with Food: Give yourself permission to eat all types of foods without guilt. Avoid labeling foods as "good" or "bad." Allow for a balanced and varied diet.

Honoring Cravings: Allow yourself to enjoy the foods you crave. Deprivation can lead to overeating or feelings of guilt. Savoring your favorite foods in moderation is a part of intuitive eating.

Respecting Your Body: Accept and appreciate your body for what it is. Focus on what your body can do rather than conforming to external ideals. Treat your body with respect and kindness.

Discovering Satisfaction: Seek satisfaction from your meals. Choose foods that you enjoy and that leave you feeling nourished and content.

Mindful Eating: Practice mindful eating by being fully present during meals. Engage your senses, savor the flavors, and eat without distractions.

Rejecting the Diet Mentality: Let go of the diet mentality and the concept of strict food rules. Focus on nourishing your body instead of following external guidelines.

Embracing Body Diversity: Recognize and celebrate the diversity of body shapes and sizes. Let go of the pursuit of an idealized body and embrace your own unique physique.

Honoring Your Feelings Without Using Food: Acknowledge and address your emotions without turning to food for comfort. Find alternative ways to cope with stress and emotional challenges

Honor Your Health: Make food choices that honor your health and well-being. Focus on overall nourishment rather than rigid dietary rules.
Intuitive eating is a personalized journey that involves reconnecting with your body and cultivating a positive relationship with food. It's about embracing a flexible and sustainable approach to eating that prioritizes well-being and self-compassion.

STRESS MANAGEMENT FOR GUT HEALTH

Stress management is crucial for maintaining gut health, as there is a strong connection between the brain and the gut. Chronic stress can negatively impact digestion and contribute to various gastrointestinal issues. Here are stress management strategies to support gut health:

1. Mindfulness Meditation:
Practice mindfulness meditation to bring your attention to the present moment. This can help reduce stress and promote a calm state of mind, positively impacting gut function.

2. Deep Breathing Exercises:
Engage in deep breathing exercises to activate the body's relaxation response. Deep, diaphragmatic breathing can help calm the nervous system and alleviate stress.

3. Yoga:
Regular yoga practice combines physical movement with mindfulness, promoting relaxation and reducing stress. Certain yoga poses may specifically target the digestive system.

4. Progressive Muscle Relaxation (PMR):
PMR consists of systematically tensing and then relaxing various muscle groups.. This technique helps release physical tension and can be beneficial for stress-induced gut issues.

5. Regular Exercise:
Incorporate regular physical activity into your routine. Exercise has been shown to reduce stress hormones and positively impact gut health.

6. Journaling:
Keep a stress journal to identify and manage sources of stress. Writing down your thoughts and feelings can provide clarity and help you develop effective coping strategies.

7. Social Support:
Maintain strong social connections. Talking to friends, family, or a support network can provide emotional support and reduce feelings of isolation or stress.

8. Prioritize Sleep:
Ensure you get sufficient, quality sleep. Sleep deprivation can make stress worse and have a detrimental effect on gut health. Establish a consistent sleep routine for better overall well-being.

9. Limit Caffeine and Alcohol:
Excessive caffeine and alcohol consumption can contribute to stress and negatively affect the gut. Moderation is key for these substances.

10. Healthy Nutrition: Consume a well-balanced diet rich in fruits, vegetables and whole grains and lean proteins. Nutrient-dense foods provide essential vitamins and minerals that support stress resilience and gut health.

11. Time Management: Effectively manage your time to reduce feelings of overwhelm.Set reasonable goals, prioritize your work, and divide difficult projects into smaller, more doable ones.

12. Cognitive Behavioral Therapy (CBT): Consider CBT, a therapeutic approach that helps to identify and modify negative thought patterns and behaviors, reducing stress and improving mental well-being

13. Nature Exposure: Spend time in nature. Whether its a walk in the park or simply enjoying green spaces. Exposure to nature has been linked to stress reduction.

14. Holistic Practices: Explore holistic practices such as acupuncture, aromatherapy or massage therapy. These complementary approaches can contribute to overall stress reduction.

15. Seek Professional Support: If stress becomes overwhelming, consider seeking support from mental health professionals. Therapy can provide tools and coping strategies to manage stress effectively.

Combining these stress management strategies with a healthy lifestyle can positively impact gut health. It's important to note that everyone's stress management needs are unique, so experiment with different techniques to find what works best for you. If gut issues persist, consult with a healthcare professional for personalized advice.

MINDFUL MEALTIME RITUALS

A mindful mealtime ritual involves intentionally bringing your full attention and awareness to the act of eating. It is about being present in the moment and savoring the experience of your meal without distractions. This practice draws from mindfulness, which is the cultivation of a heightened and non-judgmental awareness of the present moment.

Key components of a mindful mealtime ritual include:

Conscious Preparation: Take the time to prepare your meal with care and attention. Engage with the ingredients and cooking process, appreciating the effort that goes into creating a nourishing meal.

Gratitude: Start your meal with a moment of gratitude. Express thanks for the food on your plate, considering the effort of those involved in its production and preparation.

Setting the Scene: Create a pleasant and conducive environment for eating. Set the table thoughtfully, use appealing tableware, and perhaps incorporate elements like candles or soft music to enhance the dining experience.

Mindful Breathing: Before starting to eat, take a few deep breaths to center yourself and bring your focus to the present moment. This helps clear your mind of distractions and sets the tone for a mindful meal.

Sensory Awareness: Engage your senses fully during the meal. Note the colors, textures, and aromas of the food. Chew slowly and savor the flavors. This sensory awareness deepens your connection to the experience.

Elimination of Distractions: Turn off electronic devices and avoid multitasking. Eating without distractions allows you to fully concentrate on the act of eating and enhances the enjoyment of your meal.

Mindful Eating: Pay attention to the process of eating itself. Chew your food thoroughly, and be aware of the sensations and tastes. Mindful eating involves being in tune with your body's hunger and fullness cues.

Appreciation for the Source: Reflect on where your food comes from, the journey it took to reach your plate, and the interconnectedness of the food system. This reflection fosters a greater appreciation for the resources involved in providing your meals.

Closing Reflection: Conclude your meal with a moment of reflection. How do you feel after eating? What did you enjoy about the meal? This reflection helps to bring closure to the eating experience.

By incorporating these elements into your mealtime routine, you can turn eating into a more intentional and satisfying experience, promoting a healthier relationship with food and fostering a sense of mindfulness in your daily life.

CHAPTER SIX - PROBIOTICS AND PREBIOTICS FOR WOMEN

Probiotics and prebiotics play important roles in supporting gut health, which, in turn, can have various benefits for overall well-being, including for women. Here's an overview of probiotics and prebiotics and their potential relevance for women:

Probiotics:

Definition:
Probiotics are live microorganisms, typically bacteria and yeast, that give health advantages when taken in sufficient quantities.s. They are often referred to as "good" or "friendly" bacteria because they promote a balanced microbial environment in the gut.

Benefits for Women:

Maintaining Vaginal Health: Probiotics can influence the balance of microorganisms in the vaginal area, helping to prevent or alleviate conditions such as bacterial vaginosis and yeast infections.

Urinary Tract Health: Some probiotic strains may assist in preventing urinary tract infections (UTIs) by promoting a healthy balance of bacteria in the urinary tract.

Digestive Health: Probiotics contribute to a balanced gut microbiome, aiding in digestion and nutrient absorption. They may also help manage digestive issues like irritable bowel syndrome (IBS) and inflammatory bowel diseases.

Immune System Support: A healthy gut microbiome, influenced by probiotics, is linked to a well-functioning immune system. This is important for overall health, including women's immune health.

Support During Pregnancy: Some studies suggest that probiotics may have a positive impact on gestational diabetes risk and may reduce the risk of complications during pregnancy.

Prebiotics:

Definition:
Prebiotics are non-digestible fibers or compounds that promote the growth and activity of beneficial bacteria in the gut. They help as a food source for probiotics.

Benefits for Women:

Gut Microbiome Health: Prebiotics nourish the beneficial bacteria in the gut, promoting a diverse and balanced microbiome. This, in turn, supports overall digestive health.

Hormonal Balance: Some research suggests that a healthy gut microbiome influenced by prebiotics may play a role in hormonal balance, which is particularly relevant for women's reproductive health.

Bone Health: Certain prebiotics, such as inulin, may enhance calcium absorption in the gut, potentially contributing to better bone health, which is particularly important for women, especially postmenopausal women.

Weight Management: Prebiotics may help with weight management by influencing gut bacteria associated with metabolism.

Food Sources:
Probiotics:
Common sources include yogurt, kefir, sauerkraut, kimchi, miso, and other fermented foods. Probiotic supplements are also available.

Prebiotics:
Natural sources include garlic, onions, leeks, asparagus, bananas, and whole grains. Prebiotic supplements are also available.

Important Considerations:
Diversity is Key: Aim for a diverse range of probiotic strains and prebiotic sources to promote a well-balanced gut microbiome.

Consultation: Before making significant changes to your diet or incorporating supplements, especially during pregnancy or if you have existing health conditions, it's advisable to consult with a healthcare professional.

In summary, probiotics and prebiotics can contribute to women's health by supporting gut health, which has far-reaching effects on various aspects of well-being. Including a variety of probiotic and prebiotic-rich foods in your diet can be a positive step toward promoting a healthy gut microbiome.

UNDERSTANDING GUT MICROBIOTA

Gut microbiota refers to the diverse community of microorganisms, including bacteria, viruses, fungi, and archaea, that inhabit the gastrointestinal tract, primarily the colon. The human gut microbiota is a complex ecosystem that plays a crucial role in various aspects of health, including digestion, metabolism, immune function, and even mental well-being. Understanding gut microbiota involves exploring its composition, functions, factors influencing it, and its impact on overall health.

Composition of Gut Microbiota:
Bacteria: The majority of the gut microbiota consists of bacteria. There are hundreds of different bacterial species, with the two dominant phyla being Bacteroidetes and Firmicutes.

Viruses: The gut is also home to a variety of viruses, mostly bacteriophages that infect bacteria. These viruses can influence bacterial populations.

Fungi: Fungi, including yeasts, are present in the gut in smaller quantities. Candida is an example of a common gut fungus.

Archaea: Archaea are single-celled microorganisms that are less abundant in the gut than bacteria but still play a role in the overall ecosystem.

Functions of Gut Microbiota:
Digestion and Nutrient Absorption: Gut bacteria assist in breaking down complex carbohydrates and fibers that are otherwise indigestible by the human digestive enzymes. They also contribute to the absorption of certain nutrients.

Immune System Regulation: The gut microbiota interacts with the immune system, helping to train it to distinguish between harmful and harmless substances. A balanced microbiome is essential for proper immune function.

Metabolism: Gut microbes can influence the host's metabolism, including the regulation of energy balance and storage. Imbalances in the microbiota have been linked to metabolic disorders like obesity and diabetes.

Synthesis of Vitamins: Some bacteria in the gut produce vitamins, such as B vitamins and vitamin K, which contribute to the host's overall health.

Protection Against Pathogens: A healthy gut microbiota acts as a barrier, preventing the colonization of harmful pathogens by occupying the available niches and producing substances that inhibit their growth.

Factors Influencing Gut Microbiota:
Diet: The composition of your diet significantly influences the types of microorganisms in your gut. A diet rich in fiber and diverse plant-based foods promotes a more diverse and healthy microbiome.

Antibiotics: The use of antibiotics can disrupt the balance of gut microbiota by affecting both harmful and beneficial bacteria.

Stress: Psychological stress can impact the gut-brain axis and alter the composition of the gut microbiota.

Age: The gut microbiota changes with age, with a more stable and diverse composition in adulthood.

Birth and Early Life: The mode of delivery (vaginal vs. cesarean) and early exposure to microbes during birth and breastfeeding influence the initial colonization of the infant's gut.

Impact on Health:
Digestive Health: A balanced microbiota is crucial for proper digestion and can help prevent conditions like irritable bowel syndrome (IBS) and inflammatory bowel diseases (IBD).

Immune Function: The gut microbiota plays a vital role in supporting immune system development and function, helping to protect against infections.

Metabolic Health: Imbalances in the gut microbiota have been linked to metabolic disorders such as obesity and type 2 diabetes.

Mental Health: Emerging research suggests a connection between the gut microbiota and mental health, with potential links to conditions like anxiety and depression.

Ways to Support a Healthy Gut Microbiota:
Dietary Fiber: Consuming a diet rich in fiber from fruits, vegetables, whole grains, and legumes supports the growth of beneficial bacteria.

Probiotics: Consuming foods with live, beneficial bacteria (such as yogurt and fermented foods) or taking probiotic supplements can contribute to a healthy microbiota.

Prebiotics: Including prebiotic-rich foods like garlic, onions, and bananas nourishes beneficial bacteria.

Limiting Antibiotic Use: Using antibiotics judiciously and only when necessary can help prevent disruptions to the gut microbiota.

Managing Stress: Stress management techniques, such as meditation and mindfulness, may positively influence the gut-brain axis.

Understanding and maintaining a healthy gut microbiota is an evolving area of research, and ongoing studies continue to uncover its intricate connections to overall health and well-being. Maintaining a diverse and balanced diet, avoiding unnecessary antibiotic use, managing stress, and incorporating probiotics and prebiotics can contribute to supporting a thriving gut microbiota.

INCORPORATING PROBIOTIC-RICH FOODS

Incorporating probiotic-rich foods into your diet is a great way to support a healthy gut microbiota. Probiotics are live microorganisms that offer various health benefits, especially for digestion and immune function. Here are some delicious and nutritious probiotic-rich foods to consider adding to your daily meals:

Yogurt:
- Choose unsweetened, plain yogurt with live and active cultures.
- Add fresh fruits, nuts, or seeds for added flavor and texture.
- Use yogurt in smoothies or as a base for dressings and dips.

Kefir:
- Kefir is a fermented milk drink that contains a variety of probiotic strains.
- Enjoy it on its own or blend it into smoothies for a tangy kick.
- Look for plain, unsweetened kefir for the most benefits.

Sauerkraut:
- Sauerkraut is fermented cabbage and a great source of probiotics.
- Add sauerkraut to sandwiches, salads, or as a side dish.
- Ensure it's raw and unpasteurized for live cultures.

Kimchi:
- Kimchi is a Korean fermented dish, usually made with cabbage and other vegetables.
- Use kimchi as a flavorful side dish or incorporate it into rice bowls and wraps.

Miso:

- Miso is a fermented soybean paste often used in Japanese cuisine.
- Make miso soup or use miso paste as a flavorful base for marinades and dressings.

Tempeh:

- Tempeh is a fermented soybean product with a firm texture and nutty flavor.
- Cook tempeh as a meat substitute in stir-fries, sandwiches, or salads.

Pickles (Brine-Cured):

- Pickles that are brine-cured (not vinegar-pickled) can be a source of probiotics.
- Enjoy pickles as a snack or add them to sandwiches and salads.

Greek Yogurt:

- Greek yogurt is strained yogurt with a thicker consistency and higher protein content.
- Use it as a creamy topping for fruits, granola, or savory dishes.

Buttermilk:

- Traditional buttermilk (cultured buttermilk) contains probiotics.
- Use it in baking, dressings, or enjoy it as a refreshing beverage.

Natto:

- Natto is a Japanese dish gotten from fermented soybeans.
- Mix natto with soy sauce and mustard and serve it over rice for a traditional dish.

Fermented Cheeses:

- Some types of cheeses, like Gouda and cheddar, are naturally fermented and may contain probiotics.

Probiotic Supplements:

- If you find it challenging to incorporate

enough probiotic-rich foods, you can consider probiotic supplements. However, it's always best to consult with a healthcare professional before starting any supplements.

When incorporating probiotic-rich foods, aim for variety to expose your gut to different strains of beneficial bacteria. Additionally, pay attention to food labels to ensure that the products contain live and active cultures. Including these foods in your diet can contribute to a diverse and healthy gut microbiota, supporting overall digestive health and well-being.

PREBIOTIC POWER FOR A HAPPY GUT

Prebiotics are non-digestible fibers and compounds that serve as food for the beneficial bacteria in your gut. By promoting the growth and activity of these good bacteria, prebiotics contribute to a healthy and balanced gut microbiota. Here are some prebiotic-rich foods to incorporate into your diet for a happy gut:

Chicory Root:
- A good source of inulin, a type of prebiotic fiber.
- Add roasted chicory root to your coffee or brew chicory root tea.

Jerusalem Artichoke:
- High in inulin and fiber.
- Steam or roast Jerusalem artichokes as a side dish or add them to salads.

Garlic:
- Contains inulin and fructooligosaccharides (FOS).
- Use fresh garlic in cooking or add it to dressings and sauces.

Onions:
- Rich in inulin and FOS.

- Include raw or cooked onions in salads, stir-fries, and various dishes.

Leeks:
- Contain inulin and fiber.
- Use leeks in soups, stews, or as a flavorful addition to various recipes.

Asparagus:
- A good source of inulin.
- Grill, roast, or steam asparagus as a side dish or add it to salads.

Bananas:
- Provide resistant starch, a type of prebiotic.
- Enjoy ripe bananas as a snack or add them to smoothies.

Oats:
- Contain beta-glucans, a type of prebiotic fiber.
- Start your day with a bowl of oatmeal or incorporate oats into baking.

Apples:
- Rich in pectin, a prebiotic fiber.
- Eat apples with the skin on as a snack or add them to salads.

Barley:
- Contains beta-glucans and soluble fiber.
- Use barley in soups, stews, or as a base for grain bowls.

Dandelion Greens:
- High in inulin and fiber.
- Add dandelion greens to salads or use them in smoothies.

Flaxseeds:
- Provide fiber and alpha-linolenic acid.
- Sprinkle ground flaxseeds on yogurt, cereal, or include them in smoothies.

Cocoa:
- Contains flavonoids and fibers that act as prebiotics.
- Enjoy dark chocolate or add cocoa

powder to smoothies and desserts.
Seaweed:
- Rich in fiber, including alginate.
- Include seaweed in salads, soups, or as a side dish.

Legumes (Lentils, Chickpeas, Beans):
- Good sources of resistant starch and fiber.
- Incorporate legumes into salads, stews, or as a protein source in various dishes.

When incorporating prebiotic-rich foods into your diet, aim for a variety of sources to provide different types of fibers to nourish diverse gut bacteria. Including these foods regularly can contribute to a happy and balanced gut microbiota, supporting overall digestive health and well-being. Additionally, staying hydrated and maintaining a balanced diet with a mix of prebiotics and probiotics can further enhance gut health.

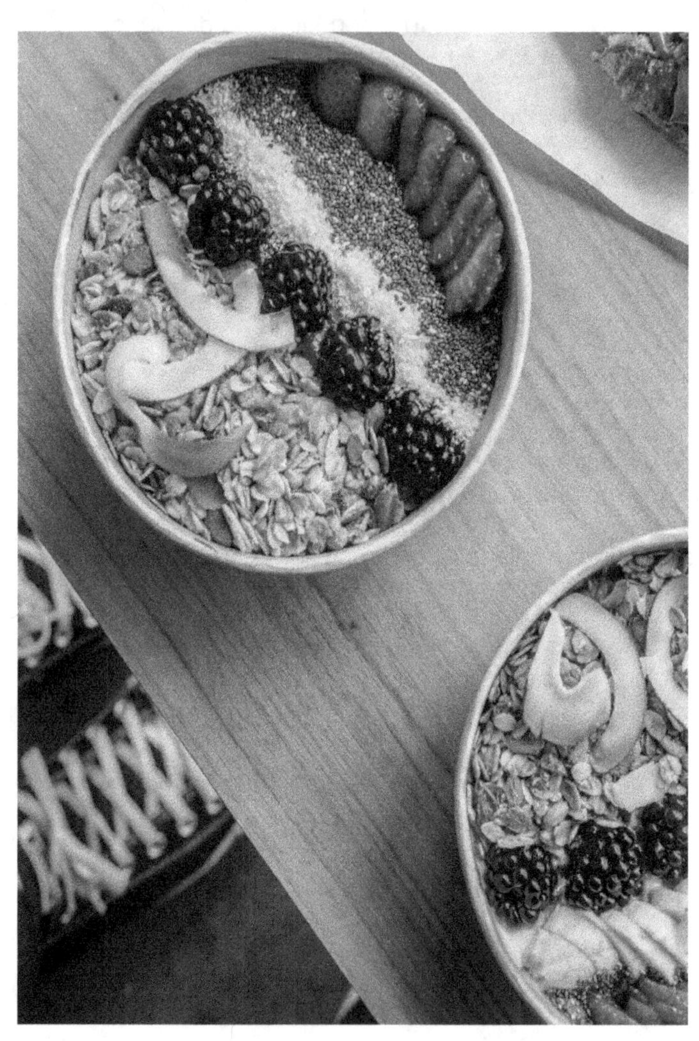

CHAPTER SEVEN - LIFESTYLE HABITS FOR GUT HARMONY

Promoting gut harmony involves adopting lifestyle habits that support the health and balance of your gut microbiota. Here are some lifestyle practices that contribute to a healthy gut:

Diverse and Balanced Diet:

Consume a variety of fruits, vegetables, whole grains, legumes, and lean proteins to provide a wide range of nutrients and fibers that nourish different types of gut bacteria.

Prebiotic-Rich Foods:

Include prebiotic-rich foods like garlic, onions, bananas, asparagus, and oats to feed and support the growth of beneficial gut bacteria.

Probiotic-Rich Foods:

Incorporate fermented foods such as yogurt, kefir, sauerkraut, kimchi, and miso into your diet to introduce beneficial live cultures to your gut.

Stay Hydrated:

Drink plenty of water to support overall digestion and maintain the mucosal lining of the intestines.

Limit Processed Foods:

Minimize the intake of highly processed and sugary foods, as they may negatively impact the diversity and balance of the gut microbiota.

Moderate Alcohol Consumption:

Limit alcohol intake, as excessive alcohol consumption can disrupt the gut microbiota.

Regular Exercise:

Engage in regular physical activity, as exercise has been associated with a more diverse and beneficial gut microbiota.

Adequate Sleep:

Prioritize quality sleep, as poor sleep patterns can affect the composition and function of the gut microbiota.

Manage Stress:

Practice stress management techniques such as meditation, deep breathing, yoga, or mindfulness to positively impact the gut-brain axis.

Avoid Overuse of Antibiotics:

Use antibiotics judiciously and only when prescribed by a healthcare professional to prevent disruptions to the gut microbiota.

Fiber-Rich Diet:

Ensure an adequate intake of dietary fiber from whole foods, as fiber promotes the growth of beneficial gut bacteria and supports regular bowel movements.

Mindful Eating:

Eat slowly, chew your food thoroughly, and pay attention to hunger and fullness cues. Mindful eating can positively influence digestion and nutrient absorption.

Regular Bowel Movements:

Establish and maintain regular bowel habits. Consistent and comfortable bowel movements contribute to gut health.

Maintain a Healthy Weight:

Aim for a healthy weight through a balanced diet and regular exercise, as obesity has been linked to alterations in the gut microbiota.

Limit Artificial Sweeteners:

Some artificial sweeteners may affect the composition and function of the gut microbiota, so moderate their consumption.

Remember that everyone's gut microbiota is unique, and individual responses to lifestyle changes may vary. It's always a good idea to make gradual adjustments and consult with a healthcare professional, especially if you have specific health concerns or conditions. Adopting these lifestyle habits can contribute to gut harmony, supporting not only digestive health but also overall well-being.

EXERCISE AND GUT HEALTH

Exercise has been shown to have positive effects on gut health, influencing the composition and diversity of the gut microbiota. Here are some ways in which exercise can contribute to a healthier gut:

Increased Microbial Diversity:

Regular physical activity correlates with a more diversified gut microbiome. A diverse microbiota is generally considered a sign of a healthy and resilient gut.

Enhanced Gut Barrier Function:

Exercise has been linked to improved gut barrier function. A strong and intact gut barrier helps prevent the entry of harmful substances into the bloodstream and maintains a healthy balance in the gut.

Reduced Inflammation:

Chronic inflammation in the gut is associated with various gastrointestinal disorders. Regular exercise has anti-inflammatory effects, which may contribute to a more balanced and healthier gut environment.

Improved Gut Motility:

Exercise can enhance gut motility, promoting regular bowel movements. This is important for preventing constipation and maintaining overall digestive health.

Increased Short-Chain Fatty Acids (SCFAs):

SCFAs are compounds produced by certain gut bacteria during the fermentation of dietary fibers. These compounds have anti-inflammatory properties and contribute to overall gut health. Regular exercise has been associated with increased SCFA production.

Positive Impact on Gut Hormones:

Exercise influences the release of hormones that can affect the gut, such as ghrelin and glucagon-like peptide-1 (GLP-1). These hormones play a role in appetite regulation and digestion.

Weight Management:

Maintaining a healthy weight through regular exercise can positively impact gut health. Obesity is associated with changes in the gut microbiota, and weight loss through exercise may help restore a healthier microbial balance.

Stress Reduction:

Exercise is a well-known stress reliever, and stress can impact the gut-brain axis. By reducing stress, exercise may indirectly contribute to a healthier gut environment.

Altered Microbial Composition:

Different types of exercise may influence the abundance of specific microbial species. For example, endurance exercise and resistance training may have distinct effects on the gut microbiota.

Post-Exercise Nutrient Utilization:

After exercise, the body may have increased nutrient uptake, which can impact the availability of nutrients in the gut, influencing microbial populations.

It's important to note that individual responses to exercise can vary, and other lifestyle factors, such as diet, also play a crucial role in shaping the gut microbiota. The most significant benefits to gut health are likely to come from a combination of regular physical activity and a balanced, fiber-rich diet.

As with any lifestyle change, it's advisable to start gradually and choose activities that you enjoy. If you have specific health concerns or conditions, it's recommended to consult with a healthcare professional or a fitness expert before making significant changes to your exercise routine.

SLEEP AS A GUT SUPPORTER

Quality sleep plays a crucial role in supporting overall health, and it has notable implications for gut health as well. Here's how sleep acts as a supporter for a healthy gut:

Circadian Rhythms and Gut Health:

The body's internal clock, or circadian rhythms, influences various physiological processes, including those in the gut. Disruptions to circadian rhythms, such as irregular sleep patterns, may impact the gut microbiota and its functions.

Gut-Brain Axis Regulation:

Adequate sleep helps regulate the gut-brain axis, a bidirectional communication system between the gut and the brain. This communication system influences various aspects of gastrointestinal function, including motility and secretion.

Reduced Inflammation:

Chronic sleep deprivation has been associated with increased inflammation, and inflammation can affect the balance of the gut microbiota. Quality sleep helps manage inflammation, supporting a healthier gut environment.

Balanced Appetite Hormones:

Hormones like ghrelin and leptin that are linked to appetite are influenced by sleep.. Inadequate sleep can lead to imbalances in these hormones, potentially contributing to overeating and changes in gut function.

Glycemic Control:

Poor sleep has been linked to impaired glucose metabolism and insulin sensitivity. Maintaining stable blood sugar levels is important for gut health, as fluctuations can impact the gut microbiota.

Restoration and Repair:

During deep sleep stages, the body undergoes repair and restoration processes. This includes the repair of gastrointestinal tissues, which is crucial for maintaining a healthy gut lining.

Microbial Balance:

Sleep patterns may influence the balance of gut bacteria. Disruptions to the sleep-wake cycle, such as shift work or irregular sleep schedules, have been associated with changes in the gut microbiota composition.

Enhanced Immune Function:

Quality sleep supports a robust immune system, and a healthy immune system is vital for maintaining gut health. Adequate rest helps the body defend against infections and maintain the balance of immune responses in the gut.

Stress Reduction:

Sleep plays a role in stress reduction, and chronic stress can impact gut health. Adequate rest helps manage stress levels, supporting a healthier gut-brain axis.

Prevention of Gut Disorders:

Chronic sleep disturbances have been linked to an increased risk of gastrointestinal disorders such as irritable bowel syndrome (IBS) and inflammatory bowel disease (IBD).

To support gut health through better sleep:

Keep a Regular Sleep Schedule: To keep your body's internal clock in check, go to bed and wake up at the same time every day.

Establish a Calm Bedtime Schedule: Set up relaxing routines before going to bed to let your body know it's time to relax.

Optimize Sleep Environment: Ensure your bedroom is conducive to sleep – cool, dark, and quiet.

Limit Stimulants: Steer clear of big meals right before bedtime and cut back on caffeine.

Frequent Exercise: Get moving on a regular basis, but steer clear of strenuous exercise right before bed.

Limit Screen Time: Reduce exposure to screens before

bedtime as the blue light emitted can interfere with melatonin production.

Manage Stress: Practice relaxation techniques such as deep breathing, meditation, or gentle yoga to manage stress levels.

Prioritizing quality sleep is a holistic approach to supporting overall well-being, including the health of the gut. If sleep issues persist, it's advisable to consult with a healthcare professional for personalized guidance and support.

BALANCING WORK AND LIFE FOR DIGESTIVE WELLBEING

Balancing work and life is essential for overall well-being, including digestive health. The demands of a busy work life, stress, and irregular schedules can have a significant impact on the digestive system. Here are some strategies to achieve a better balance and support digestive well-being:

1. Establish Regular Eating Habits:
Consistent Meal Times: Try to eat meals at regular times each day to help regulate your body's internal clock.

Avoid Skipping Meals: Skipping meals can disrupt your digestive routine. Plan and prioritize your meals, even during busy workdays.

2. Choose Nutrient-Rich Foods:
Balanced Diet: Include a variety of vegetables, whole grains, lean proteins, fruits, and healthy fats in your meal.

Hydration: Stay well-hydrated by drinking plenty of water throughout the day, as proper hydration is crucial for digestion.

3. Mindful Eating Practices:
Eat Without Distractions: Whenever possible, avoid working or watching screens while eating. Focus on the sensory experience of your food.

Chew Thoroughly: Chew your food slowly and thoroughly to aid digestion and promote a feeling of satiety.

4. Stress Management:
Regular Breaks: Take short breaks during the workday to stretch, practice deep breathing, or go for a short walk to reduce stress.

Mindfulness and Meditation: Incorporate mindfulness or meditation practices to manage stress levels and promote relaxation.

5. Work-Life Boundaries:
Set Boundaries: Establish clear boundaries between work and personal time. Limit bringing work-related stress into your personal life.

Disconnect: Create a routine for disconnecting from work emails and tasks during non-working hours.

6. Regular Physical Activity:
Exercise Routine: Make regular exercise a part of your daily schedule.. Exercise helps reduce stress, supports a healthy weight, and aids digestion.

Desk Exercises: Incorporate simple stretches or exercises, especially if you have a sedentary job.

7. Adequate Sleep:
Make sleep a priority. Aim for seven to nine hours of good sleep every night. Create a calming nighttime ritual to enhance the quality of your sleep.

Consistent Sleep Schedule: Maintain a consistent sleep schedule, even on weekends, to regulate your body's circadian rhythms.

8. Hygiene Practices:
Hand Hygiene: Practice good hand hygiene to reduce the risk of infections that can affect digestive health.

Healthy Work Environment: Maintain a clean and comfortable workspace to promote overall well-being.

9. Supportive Supplements:
Probiotics: Consider incorporating probiotic supplements to support a healthy balance of gut bacteria, especially during times of stress or when taking antibiotics.

Fiber Supplements: If necessary, include fiber supplements to support regular bowel movements.

10. Regular Health Check-ups:
Preventive Care: Schedule regular health check-ups to monitor your overall health and address any concerns related to digestion.

Balancing work and life is an ongoing process that requires attention and conscious effort. Prioritizing self-care and adopting healthy habits can significantly contribute to digestive well-being and overall vitality. If digestive issues persist, it's advisable to consult with a healthcare professional for personalized guidance and support

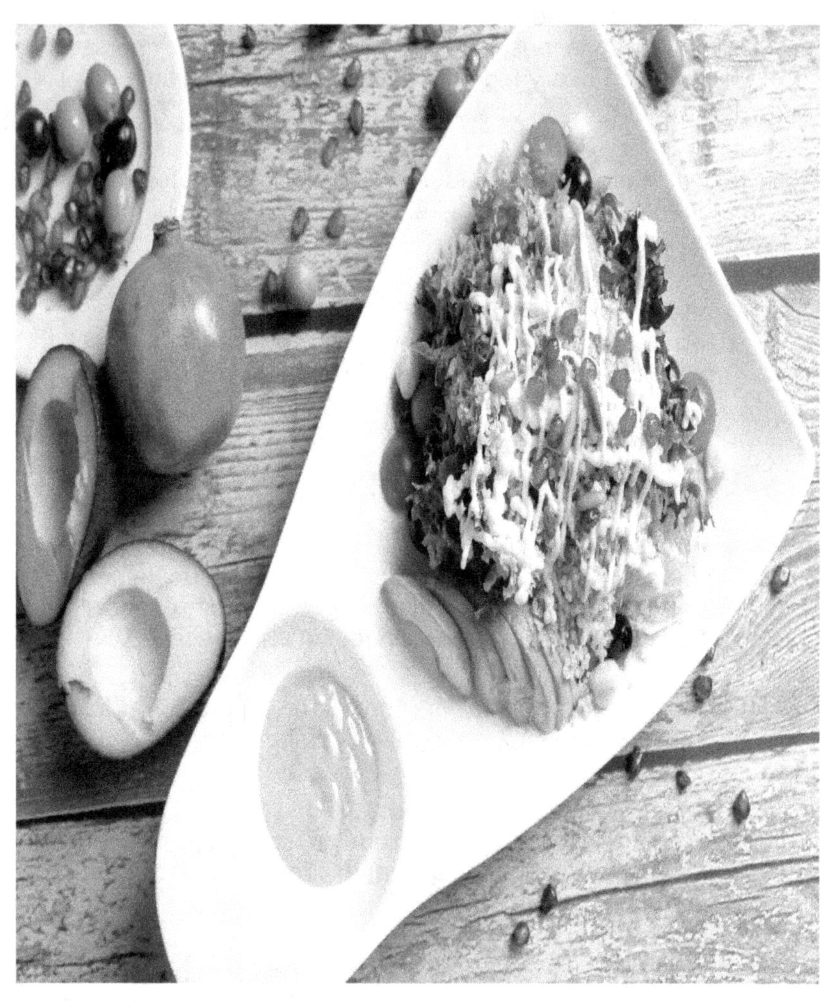

CHAPTER EIGHT - TAILORED WELLNESS FOR WOMEN

"Tailored wellness for women" generally refers to personalized approaches and strategies for promoting health and well-being that specifically cater to the unique needs and considerations of women. Women's health is a broad and diverse field that encompasses physical, mental, and emotional aspects. Here are some key areas and considerations for tailored wellness for women:

Reproductive Health: Menstrual Health: Understanding and managing menstrual cycles, addressing issues such as irregular periods, pain, or other related concerns.

Pregnancy and Postpartum: Providing support and guidance during pregnancy, childbirth, and the postpartum period.

Hormonal Balance: Addressing hormonal fluctuations throughout various life stages, including puberty, the menstrual cycle, pregnancy, perimenopause, and menopause.

Nutrition and Diet: Tailoring nutritional advice to meet the specific needs of women, considering factors such as pregnancy, lactation, and potential nutrient deficiencies.

Fitness and Exercise: Developing exercise routines that align with women's health goals and account for different life stages and fitness levels.

Mental and Emotional Well-being: Recognizing and addressing mental health concerns, including stress, anxiety, depression, and body image issues.

Providing support for life transitions and challenges

unique to women.

Preventive Care: Emphasizing regular screenings and check-ups for conditions like breast cancer, cervical cancer, and osteoporosis.

Sleep Health: Addressing sleep-related issues, which may be influenced by hormonal changes, stress, or lifestyle factors.

Sexual Health: Promoting safe and enjoyable sexual experiences.

Offering information and resources for contraception and family planning.

Community and Social Support: Creating supportive communities that address women's health concerns and foster connection and empowerment.

Education and Empowerment: Providing education on women's health issues to empower women to make informed decisions about their well-being.

Tailored wellness for women should be individualized, considering factors such as age, genetics, lifestyle, and personal preferences. It's important for women to collaborate with healthcare professionals to create a holistic and personalized wellness plan that addresses their unique needs. Additionally, staying informed about the latest research and advancements in women's health can contribute to making well-informed decisions about one's health and well-being.

AGE SPECIFIC CONSIDERATIONS

Age-specific considerations are crucial in tailoring wellness approaches to address the unique needs and challenges individuals face at different stages of life. Here's a breakdown of age-specific considerations for women's wellness:

Childhood and Adolescence:

Nutrition and Growth: Ensuring proper nutrition for growth and development.

Physical Activity: Encouraging regular exercise and promoting a healthy body image.

Puberty Education: Providing information about puberty, menstrual health, and emotional well-being.

Reproductive Years:

Menstrual Health: Addressing menstrual cycle irregularities and discomfort.

Pregnancy Planning: Providing guidance on family planning, prenatal care, and fertility awareness.

Preventive Care: Encouraging regular screenings for reproductive health, including Pap smears and mammograms.

Pregnancy and Postpartum:

Prenatal Care: Ensuring proper nutrition, monitoring health, and addressing pregnancy-related concerns.

Postpartum Recovery: Supporting mental and physical

well-being during the postpartum period.

Adulthood (20s to 40s):

Career and Family Balance: Balancing work and family responsibilities.

Mental Health: Addressing stress, anxiety, and depression.

Nutrition and Exercise: Maintaining a healthy lifestyle to prevent chronic diseases.

Perimenopause (Late 30s to Early 50s):

Hormonal Changes: Managing symptoms associated with perimenopause.

Bone Health: Addressing bone density and osteoporosis prevention.

Heart Health: Paying attention to cardiovascular health.

Menopause and Beyond (50s and Beyond):

Hormonal Changes: Managing symptoms of menopause and considering hormone replacement therapy if appropriate.

Bone Health: Continued focus on bone density and osteoporosis prevention.

Cardiovascular Health: Monitoring heart health and addressing risks associated with aging.

Senior Years (65 and Beyond):

Cognitive Health: Addressing cognitive decline and promoting brain health.

Bone and Joint Health: Managing arthritis and other age-related conditions.

Social Connections: Encouraging social engagement and community involvement for mental well-being.

End of Life Considerations:

Palliative Care: Focusing on comfort and quality of life.

Healthcare Decisions: Discussing and documenting end-of-life preferences.

Tailoring wellness for women at different life stages involves recognizing the evolving needs and priorities associated with aging. Regular check-ups, age-appropriate screenings, and open communication with healthcare providers play essential roles in promoting women's health across the lifespan.

PREGNANCY AND POSTPARTUM GUT CARE

Pregnancy and postpartum gut care are essential aspects of women's health during and after childbirth. Maintaining a healthy gut is crucial for overall well-being, as it can impact digestion, nutrient absorption, and immune function. Here are some considerations for pregnancy and postpartum gut care:

Pregnancy Gut Care:

Balanced Nutrition: Consume a well-balanced diet rich in fiber, fruits, vegetables, whole grains, and lean proteins to support gut health.

Probiotics: Include foods high in probiotics, such as kefir, sauerkraut, kimchi, and yogurt, to help maintain a balanced population of gut bacteria.

Hydration: Stay adequately hydrated to support digestion and prevent constipation, a common issue during pregnancy.

Supplements: Discuss with your healthcare provider about the need for prenatal vitamins or other supplements that may support gut and overall health.

Fiber Intake: Include fiber in your diet to prevent constipation. Foods like whole grains, legumes, and fruits can be beneficial.

Regular Exercise: Engage in moderate exercise to promote healthy digestion and overall well-being.

Postpartum Gut Care:

Postpartum Nutrition: Continue to focus on a nutrient-dense diet that supports recovery and breastfeeding if applicable.

Probiotics: Consider continuing to incorporate probiotic-rich foods or supplements to aid in gut health, especially if you are breastfeeding.

Hydration: Stay well-hydrated to support breastfeeding and overall health.

Gradual Resumption of Exercise: Ease back into

physical activity to support digestion and energy levels. Before starting any exercise routine, consult with your healthcare provider.

Fiber-Rich Foods: Continue to include fiber in your diet to prevent constipation and support gut health.

Mindful Eating: Practice mindful eating, paying attention to hunger and fullness cues, which can positively impact digestion.

Addressing Digestive Issues: If you experience digestive discomfort or issues, consult with your healthcare provider for guidance.

Balancing Hormones: Understand the impact of hormonal changes on gut health and work with your healthcare provider to address any concerns.

Self-Care: Prioritize self-care to manage stress, which can influence gut health.

Always consult with your healthcare provider before making significant changes to your diet, exercise routine, or supplementation during pregnancy and postpartum. They can offer tailored guidance according to your particular health requirements and situations. Additionally, each woman's experience during and after pregnancy is unique, so it's essential to tailor gut care strategies to your specific situation.

MENOPAUSE AND BEYOND

Menopause marks the end of a woman's reproductive years and is typically defined as the cessation of menstrual periods for 12 consecutive months. The transition through menopause and the postmenopausal years bring about various hormonal, physical, and emotional changes.

Gut care during menopause and beyond is important for maintaining overall health and well-being. The hormonal changes associated with menopause can influence digestive health, and aging itself can bring about changes in the gastrointestinal system. Here are some considerations for gut care during menopause and beyond:

1. Nutrient-Rich Diet: Consume a well-balanced diet rich in fiber, fruits, vegetables, whole grains, lean proteins, and healthy fats. Adequate nutrition is crucial for supporting overall health, including gut function.

2. Probiotics and Prebiotics: Incorporate probiotic-rich foods (e.g., yogurt, kefir, sauerkraut, kimchi) to support the balance of gut bacteria. Prebiotics, found in foods like garlic, onions, and bananas, can also help nourish beneficial gut microbes.

3. Hydration: Stay well-hydrated to support digestion and prevent constipation, which may become more common during menopause.

4. Bone Health and Calcium: Focus on maintaining bone health, which is crucial during and after menopause. Add foods high in calcium, such as dairy, leafy greens, and fortified meals.

5. Fiber Intake: Ensure an adequate intake of dietary fiber to promote regular bowel movements and support a healthy gut. Whole grains, legumes, fruits, and vegetables are examples of foods high in fiber.

6. Mindful Eating: Practice mindful eating to support healthy digestion. Chew food thoroughly and pay attention to hunger and fullness cues.

7. Hormone Replacement Therapy (HRT) Considerations: If undergoing hormone replacement therapy, discuss potential digestive side effects with your healthcare provider. Hormonal changes can impact the gastrointestinal system.

8. Regular Exercise: Engage in regular physical activity to support overall health and digestion. Exercise can help alleviate symptoms such as bloating and constipation.

9. Manage Stress: Chronic stress can affect gut health. Engage in stress-relieving activities like yoga, meditation, and deep breathing.

10. Regular Check-ups: Schedule regular check-ups with your healthcare provider to address any digestive issues or concerns. Gut health is interconnected with overall health, and any persistent symptoms should be evaluated.

11. Supplements: Consider supplements if needed, such as fiber supplements or probiotics. Before adding any new supplements to your routine, consult with your healthcare provider.

12. Individualized Approach: Menopausal experiences vary, so it's important to tailor gut care strategies to your specific needs. Consult with healthcare professionals for personalized advice.

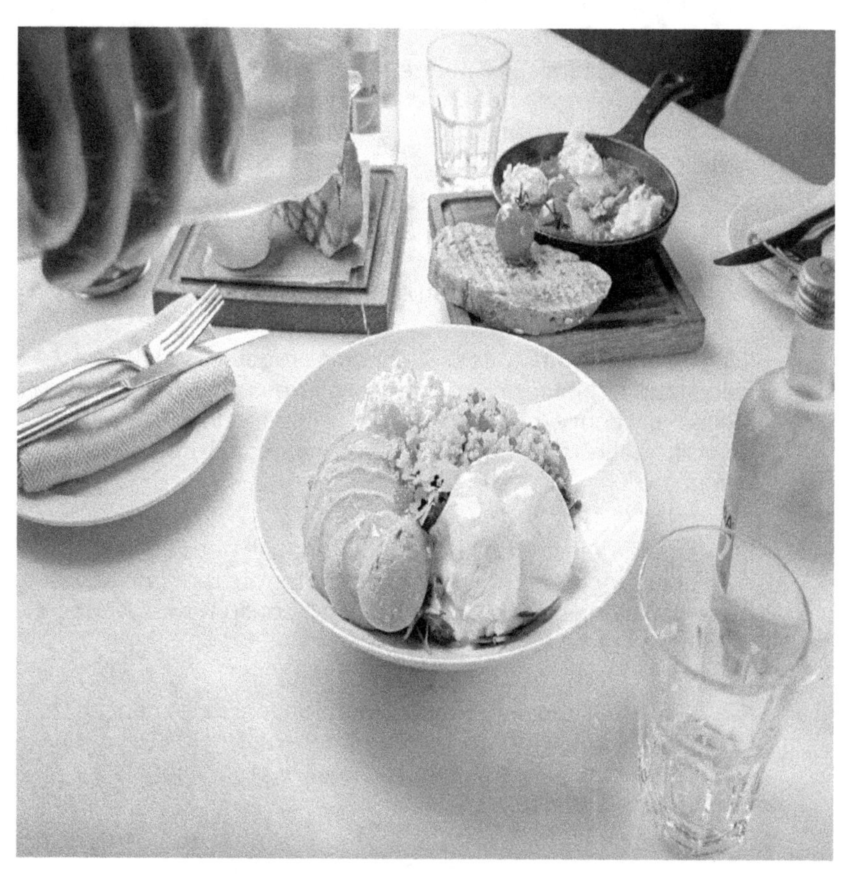

CHAPTER NINE - CRAFTING YOUR PERSONAL MEAL TIME

Crafting a personalized meal plan to support gut health involves incorporating a variety of nutrient-dense foods that promote a balanced and diverse microbiome. Here are general guidelines to help you create a meal plan focused on gut health:

1. Diverse, Fiber-Rich Vegetables:
Include a Rainbow of Vegetables: Aim for a variety of colorful vegetables to provide a range of nutrients and fibers that nourish different types of gut bacteria.

Leafy Greens: Incorporate leafy greens like spinach, kale, and Swiss chard, which are rich in fiber and other essential nutrients.

2. Fruits:
Choose Whole Fruits: Opt for whole fruits, such as berries, apples, and citrus fruits, which contain fiber and beneficial antioxidants.

Prebiotic Fruits: Include fruits with prebiotic fibers, like bananas, garlic, and onions, to support the growth of beneficial bacteria.

3. Whole Grains:
Quinoa, Brown Rice, and Oats: Choose whole grains that provide fiber and essential nutrients. These grains can contribute to a healthy gut environment.

4. Lean Proteins:
Fish and Poultry: Include fatty fish for omega-3 fatty acids, and lean poultry for protein.

Plant-Based Proteins: Incorporate plant-based protein sources such as legumes, lentils, and beans.

5. Fermented Foods:
Yogurt: Choose plain, unsweetened yogurt with live cultures for probiotics.

Kefir: Include kefir, a fermented milk drink that is rich in probiotics.

Sauerkraut, Kimchi, and Miso: Add fermented vegetables and soy products for additional probiotic diversity.

6. Healthy Fats:
Avocado: Rich in monounsaturated fats and fiber.

Nuts and Seeds: Provide healthy fats, fiber, and various nutrients.

7. Prebiotic Foods:
Garlic and Onions: Include these aromatic vegetables, known for their prebiotic properties.

Asparagus and Leeks: Add these vegetables to support the growth of beneficial bacteria.

8. Hydration:
Water: Stay well-hydrated, as water is essential for digestion and overall health.

Herbal Teas: Consider herbal teas, such as ginger or peppermint, which may have digestive benefits.

9. Limit Processed Foods and Added Sugars:
Minimize Processed Foods: Limit processed and highly refined foods, which may negatively impact gut health.

Reduce Added Sugars: High sugar intake can affect the balance of gut bacteria.

10. Proper Portion Control:
Balanced Meals: Aim for balanced meals with a mix of macronutrients (carbohydrates, proteins, and fats).

Regular Eating Schedule: Maintain a regular eating schedule to support digestion.

11. Experiment and Listen to Your Body:
Food Journaling: Keep a food journal to track how different foods affect your digestion and overall well-being.

Intuitive Eating: Listen to your body's signals and adjust your meal plan based on how you feel after eating certain foods.

12. Consult with a Registered Dietitian or Healthcare Professional:
Individualized Guidance: Seek personalized advice from a registered dietitian or healthcare professional to tailor your meal plan to your specific needs and health conditions.

Remember, everyone's digestive system is unique, so it may take some experimentation to find the foods that work best for you. If you have specific health concerns or conditions, it's crucial to consult with a healthcare professional or a registered dietitian for personalized guidance.

BUILDING A WHOLESOME SUPER GUTS MEAL PLAN

Creating a meal plan for a wholesome and super gut-friendly diet involves incorporating foods that promote a healthy and diverse microbiome. Here's a sample meal plan to support optimal gut health:

Breakfast:

Greek Yogurt Parfait:

- Ingredients:
    - Greek yogurt (probiotic-rich)
    - Mixed berries (prebiotic)
    - Chia seeds (fiber)
    - Almond slices (healthy fats)
    - Drizzle of honey (optional)

Whole Grain Toast with Avocado:

- Ingredients:
    - Whole grain bread (fiber)
    - Mashed avocado (healthy fats)
    - Cherry tomatoes (fiber, vitamins)
    - Sprinkle of flaxseeds (fiber)

Mid-Morning Snack:
Banana and Almond Butter:

- Ingredients:
    - Banana (prebiotic)
    - Almond butter (healthy fats, protein)

Lunch:

Quinoa and Vegetable Bowl:

- Ingredients:
    - Quinoa (fiber, protein)
    - Grilled chicken or tofu (protein)
    - Steamed broccoli, carrots, and bell peppers (fiber)
    - Kimchi or sauerkraut (fermented food)

Mixed Green Salad:

- Ingredients:
  - Mixed greens (fiber)
  - Cherry tomatoes (fiber, vitamins)
  - Cucumber slices (fiber)
  - Pumpkin seeds (healthy fats)

Afternoon Snack:
Smoothie:

- Ingredients:
  - Spinach (fiber, vitamins)
  - Banana (prebiotic)
  - Blueberries (prebiotic)
  - Greek yogurt (probiotic)
  - Almond milk (nutrients, hydration)

Dinner:

Salmon with Quinoa and Roasted Vegetables:

- Ingredients:
  - Baked or grilled salmon (omega-3 fatty acids)
  - Quinoa (fiber, protein)
  - Roasted sweet potatoes, zucchini, and asparagus (fiber)
  - Garlic and olive oil for flavor (prebiotic)

Stir-Fried Tofu and Vegetables:

- Ingredients:
  - Tofu (protein)
  - Stir-fried mixed vegetables (fiber)
  - Brown rice (fiber)
  - Ginger and sesame oil for flavor (prebiotic)

Evening Snack:
Kefir Smoothie:

- Ingredients:
    - Kefir (probiotic)
    - Pineapple chunks (prebiotic)
    - Handful of almonds (healthy fats)

Tips for Super Gut Health:

Hydration:

To aid in digestion, drink lots of water throughout the day.

Variety and Color:
Include a variety of colorful fruits and vegetables to ensure a diverse range of nutrients and fiber.

Probiotics and Fermented Foods:
Incorporate yogurt, kefir, sauerkraut, kimchi, or other fermented foods regularly.
Prebiotics:
Include prebiotic-rich foods like bananas, garlic, onions, and whole grains.

Whole Foods:

Focus on whole, unprocessed foods to maximize nutrient intake.

Balanced Macronutrients:

Ensure a balance of carbohydrates, healthy fats, and proteins in each meal.

Listen to Your Body:

Pay attention to how your body responds to different foods and adjust your plan accordingly.

Remember, this is just a sample meal plan, and individual needs may vary. It's essential to tailor your diet to your specific preferences, dietary restrictions, and health conditions. If you have specific concerns or health issues, consider consulting with a registered dietitian or healthcare professional for personalized guidance.

SAMPLE MEAL PLANS FOR DIFFERENT LIFESTYLES

Here are sample meal plans designed to promote gut health, tailored for different lifestyles:

1. General Gut Health Meal Plan:
Suitable for those looking to support overall gut health.

Breakfast:

- Overnight oats with Greek yogurt, topped with mixed berries and a sprinkle of flaxseeds

Mid-Morning Snack:

- Banana with almond butter

Lunch:

- wrap made with whole grain tortilla, hummus, and mixed greens with grilled chicken or tofu
- Side of fermented vegetables (sauerkraut or kimchi)

Afternoon Snack:

- Plain, unsweetened yogurt with a handful of walnuts and a drizzle of honey

Dinner:

- Baked salmon with quinoa
- Steamed broccoli and carrots
- Miso soup

2. Vegetarian Gut Health Meal Plan:

Designed for those following a vegetarian lifestyle.

Breakfast:

- Smoothie with spinach, pineapple, banana, chia seeds, and kefir

Mid-Morning Snack:

- Apple slices with almond butter

Lunch:

- Lentil and vegetable stew with a side of brown rice
- Greek salad with olives and feta cheese

Afternoon Snack:

- Hummus with carrot and cucumber sticks

Dinner:

- Quinoa-stuffed bell peppers with black beans and corn
- Grilled zucchini on the side

3. Low-FODMAP Gut Health Meal Plan:

Suitable for individuals following a low-FODMAP diet for gut sensitivities.

Breakfast:

- Scrambled eggs with spinach and tomatoes
- Gluten-free toast with lactose-free butter

Mid-Morning Snack:

- Strawberries with lactose-free yogurt

Lunch:

- Grilled chicken or tofu with a quinoa and green bean salad
- FODMAP-friendly dressing

Afternoon Snack:

- Rice cakes with lactose-free cream cheese and sliced cucumber

Dinner:

- Baked cod with mashed potatoes (without garlic/onion)
- Steamed carrots and zucchini

4. Probiotic-Rich Gut Health Meal Plan:

Focuses on incorporating foods rich in probiotics.

Breakfast:

- Kefir smoothie with mixed berries and a tablespoon of chia seeds

Mid-Morning Snack:

- Fermented coconut yogurt with a handful of almonds

Lunch:

- Shrimp or tempeh stir-fry with bok choy, bell peppers, and ginger
- Brown rice

Afternoon Snack:

- Kimchi or sauerkraut with whole grain crackers

Dinner:

- Greek salad with grilled chicken and tzatziki dressing
- Quinoa on the side

5. Gluten-Free and Gut-Friendly Meal Plan:

For persons with gluten sensitivities or celiac disease.

Breakfast:

- Gluten-free oatmeal with almond milk, topped with sliced strawberries and pumpkin seeds

Mid-Morning Snack:

- Rice cakes with peanut butter

Lunch:

- Grilled salmon or chickpea patties with a gluten-free quinoa salad
- Steamed broccoli and carrots

Afternoon Snack:

- Gluten-free crackers with goat cheese and cherry tomatoes

Dinner:

- Turkey or tofu lettuce wraps with gluten-free soy sauce
- Stir-fried bell peppers and snap peas

These meal plans are general examples and may need adjustments based on individual preferences, dietary restrictions, and health conditions. If you have specific dietary concerns or conditions, it's advisable to consult with a healthcare professional or a registered dietitian for personalized advice.

ADAPTING MEAL PLANS TO YOUR UNIQUE NEEDS

Adapting meal plans to your unique needs involves considering your individual preferences, dietary restrictions, health goals, and lifestyle factors. Here are some general guidelines to help you customize and tailor meal plans:

1. Assess Your Dietary Preferences: Vegetarian or Vegan: If you prefer plant-based options, replace animal proteins with sources like beans, lentils, tofu, or tempeh. Low-Carb or Keto: Choose non-starchy vegetables, healthy fats, and protein sources while minimizing carbohydrate intake.

Gluten-Free: Opt for gluten-free grains, such as quinoa or rice, and choose gluten-free alternatives for bread, pasta, and other grain-based products.

2. Consider Dietary Restrictions: Lactose Intolerance: Choose lactose-free or dairy alternatives.
Nut Allergies: Substitute nuts with seeds or other protein sources.

Celiac Disease or Gluten Sensitivity: Select gluten-free grains and avoid wheat, barley, and rye products.

3. Evaluate Your Health Goals: Weight Management: Adjust portion sizes and balance macronutrients based on your calorie needs.
Heart Health: Prioritize complete meals, low-fat dairy products, and lean meats.

Blood Sugar Control: Focus on complex carbohydrates, fiber, and balanced meals to stabilize blood sugar levels.

4. Consider Meal Timing and Frequency: Intermittent Fasting: Adjust your meal plan based on your fasting and eating windows.
Small Frequent Meals: If you prefer multiple smaller meals, plan snacks between main meals.

5. Personalize Portion Sizes: Listen to Hunger Cues: Pay attention to your body's hunger and fullness signals. Adjust Portions: Modify serving sizes based on your activity level and energy needs.

6. Incorporate Variety: Explore Different Foods: Include a wide range of fruits, vegetables, proteins, and whole grains to ensure a diverse nutrient intake.
Rotate Proteins: Rotate between animal and plant-based protein sources to diversify amino acid profiles.

7. Hydration: Water Intake: Adjust your water intake based on your activity level, climate, and individual needs.

8. Mindful Eating: Mindful Habits: Practice mindful eating by savoring each bite and paying attention to hunger and fullness.
Eliminate Distractions: Minimize distractions while eating to focus on the sensory experience of your meals.

9. Consult with a Professional: Registered Dietitian or Nutritionist: If you have specific health concerns, dietary restrictions, or goals, seek guidance from a registered dietitian or nutritionist.

10. Experiment and Adjust: Trial and Error: Experiment with different foods and meal structures to find what works best for you.
Be Flexible: Be open to adjusting your plan as needed based on your body's response and feedback.

Remember, the key to a sustainable and enjoyable meal plan is finding a balance that fits your individual needs and preferences. It's always a good idea to consult with a healthcare professional or a registered dietitian for personalized guidance based on your unique health situation.

CELEBRATING YOUR JOURNEY TO WHOLESOME SUPER GUTS

Celebrating your journey to wholesome super guts is a wonderful way to acknowledge the efforts you've put into nurturing your digestive health. Here are some ideas to celebrate and honor your commitment to a healthy gut:

1. Reflect on Achievements:
   - Take a moment to reflect on the positive changes you've made in your diet and lifestyle.
   - Acknowledge any improvements in your digestion, energy levels, or overall well-being.

2. Share Your Success:
   - Share your journey with friends or family who have supported you. Celebrate together and inspire others to prioritize gut health.

3. Gut-Friendly Feast:
   - Prepare a special meal with a focus on gut-friendly foods.
   - Include fermented foods, prebiotics, and a variety of colorful, nutrient-dense ingredients.

4. Create a Wholesome Super Guts Recipe Book:
   - Compile your favorite gut-friendly recipes in a personalized recipe book.
   - Include notes on how each recipe has contributed to your well-being.

5. Mindful Eating Ritual:
  - Practice mindful eating with a special meal.
  - Take the time to savor each bite, appreciating the flavors and nourishment.

6. Self-Care Day:
  - Treat yourself to a day of self-care, focusing on relaxation and stress reduction.
  - Activities could include a massage, yoga session, or a peaceful nature walk.

7. Express Gratitude:
  - Write down things you are grateful for in your gut health journey.
  - Express gratitude for the resilience and adaptability of your body.

8. Set New Goals:
  - Consider setting new goals for continued gut health improvement.
  - These could include trying new gut-friendly foods or incorporating different forms of exercise.

9. Host a Gut Health Workshop or Gathering:
  - Share your knowledge and experiences with friends or community members.
  - Host a workshop, cooking class, or gathering to discuss the importance of gut health.

10. Connect with Others:
  - Join online communities or forums related to gut health.
  - Share your story and connect with others who are on a similar journey.

11. Celebrate with Gut-Healthy Treats:
  - Enjoy a treat that aligns with your gut-friendly

lifestyle, such as a smoothie bowl, kombucha, or a homemade fermented beverage.

12. Document Your Journey:
    - Start a journal to document your gut health journey.
    - Include thoughts, challenges, and triumphs, and revisit it periodically to see how far you've come.

13. Mind-Body Activities:
    - Engage in activities that promote mind-body connection, such as meditation or a relaxing bath.

14. Share Knowledge:
    - Educate others about the importance of gut health by sharing informative articles, books, or documentaries.

15. Celebrate Regularly:
    - Make celebrating your journey to wholesome super guts a regular practice to reinforce positive habits and sustained commitment.

Remember that your journey to gut health is unique, and celebrating milestones along the way can be a powerful motivator for continued well-being. Celebrate not only the destination but also the daily efforts and choices that contribute to your holistic health.

CONCLUSION

In conclusion, the concept of a wholesome super gut holds immense promise for women's health and well-being. Through the integration of dietary choices, lifestyle adjustments, and targeted supplements, women can cultivate a resilient and balanced gut microbiome, offering a plethora of benefits ranging from improved digestion to enhanced immunity and mental well-being.

The understanding of how the gut microbiome influences various aspects of women's health, including hormonal balance, reproductive health, and mood regulation, underscores the importance of nurturing a diverse and thriving microbial community within the gut. Adopting a diet rich in fiber, prebiotics, and probiotics, along with regular exercise and stress management, serves as foundational pillars in promoting gut health and overall vitality.

Furthermore, incorporating specific superfoods and supplements, such as fermented foods, omega-3 fatty acids, and targeted probiotic strains, can further optimize gut function and support women's unique health needs. Embracing a holistic approach to gut health empowers women to take proactive steps towards achieving optimal well-being and longevity.

As research continues to unveil the intricate connections between the gut microbiome and women's health, the significance of prioritizing gut health cannot be overstated. By nurturing a wholesome super gut, women can unlock a pathway to vitality, resilience, and vitality, enabling them to thrive in every aspect of their lives.

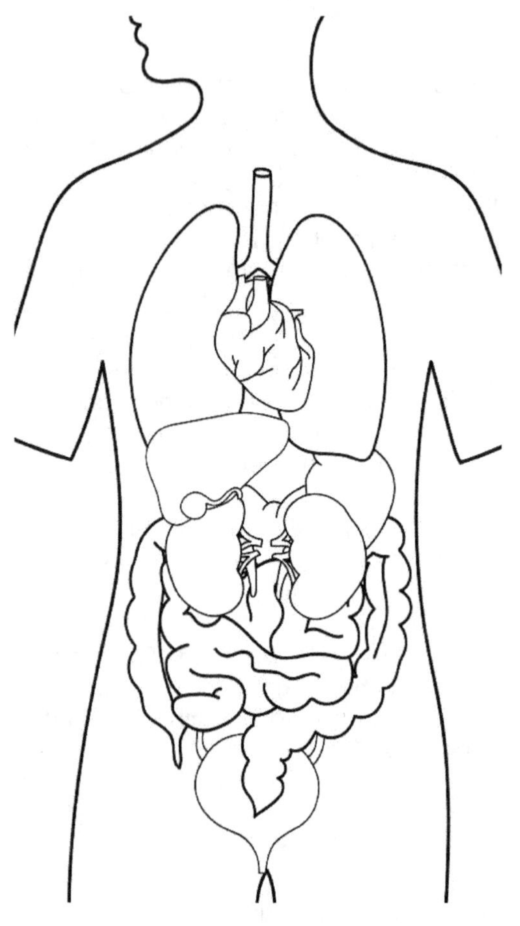